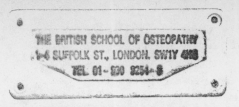
SAFE SEX

THE PLEASURES
WITHOUT THE PITFALLS

ELLIOT PHILIPP

COLUMBUS BOOKS

LONDON

First published in Great Britain in 1987 by
Columbus Books Limited
19–23 Ludgate Hill
London, EC4M 7PD

BRITISH LIBRARY CATALOGUING IN PUBLICATION DATA

Philipp, Elliot
Safe sex: the pleasures without the pitfalls
1. Contraception 2. Venereal diseases
I. Title
613.9′4   RG136

ISBN 0-86287-352-5

Typeset in Korinna by Poole Typesetting (Wessex) Ltd.,
Bournemouth
Printed and bound by Guernsey Press,
Guernsey, Channel Islands

CONTENTS

INTRODUCTION

I am confused and worried.
You are confused and worried.
He/she is confused and worried.
We are confused and worried.
They are confused and worried.
Who would not be?

Every day, everywhere we look and listen, there are posters,
warnings on radio and television, notices through the letterbox
and talk, talk, talk as well as questions and answers. Worried
questions. And confusing answers. Bishops and senior
policemen who have never examined an infected boy or a
pregnant girl sound off as though they knew all about sex, all
about morality, all about emotions and all about everything.
They presume not only to contradict one another but also to
contradict the experts who put out the posters and warnings
and notices, and who may very well know something about
human sexual behaviour.

Can we have sex? Is it safe? Am I risking pregnancy or
catching a possibly dangerous infection? Can I go to bed with
my boyfriend who has been away on holiday and had casual sex
with a girl, and says they got to know two gay boys staying at
the same hotel? Can I use the glass in a restaurant that may
have been placed on the table by who knows who? What will
happen if I prick my lip with a fork washed up by a stranger who
may have caught something? How safe or unsafe is it even to
touch people, let alone make love to them?

This book will try to provide some answers.

1
WHAT MAKES SAFE SEX
AND WHAT MAKES UNSAFE SEX?

Sex with one partner continued for a long time, giving pleasure equally to both, is not based on just being good together in bed. It inevitably involves a mental relationship, in other words a meeting of both minds and bodies, where both have respect for one another. It enriches both partners enormously and such a relationship, once started, can be the basis of a very rewarding, stable household.

Safe sex is sex that avoids all the dangers that can be associated with sexual relations. These dangers, all of which are avoidable, are:

1   Becoming pregnant. This can certainly be avoided by effective birth control (see pages 49–67).

2   Becoming infected with a sexually transmitted disease (STD). The risks of this are spelled out in the description of the diseases (see pages 68–88) and they are always increased if there have been multiple partners on either side. Even in a first sexual relationship for one person, the risks are high if it is with a partner who has had many lovers. The risks can be minimized by choosing your partner carefully and also by using certain safeguards, in particular condoms (see page 50–51). Condoms, however, are not full protection.

3   Being hurt emotionally, either by being rejected by your partner, or by having to reject your partner because you have made a bad choice. Both these may involve some loss of self-respect, and, if either of them happens too often, may result in your considering yourself next to worthless.

BECOMING PREGNANT

The link that had until recently always existed between sexual intercourse and becoming pregnant was broken, or at least very much weakened, when doctors invented oral contraception, the first really reliable birth control method in the form of a pill for women (see pages 54–57). With the pill it is safe to have intercourse without the risk of starting an unwanted pregnancy. This applies so long as the pill is taken daily for three weeks out of every four, or according to the instructions on the packet: it is an every-day pill or a 'mini-pill' if it is taken every day of every month.

There were some pretty good contraceptive methods before the pill was invented. These have not gone away and they are described in Chapter 4.

Less reliable forms of contraception were also available long before the pill – coitus interruptus and homely methods like putting a scooped-out half-lemon in the vagina. These older, less sure, methods had the great disadvantage that the couple had to interrupt love-making to use them, or even had to prepare themselves beforehand. That took a lot of the spontaneity away from the intercourse and some of the glamour as well. Worse still, the rhythm or dates method rules out love-making at all, if it is to be reasonably effective, except for a few days each month.

Then came the pill. 'Wonderful!' everybody exclaimed. 'Freedom has come. Women can be much more liberal in sexual relationships and there will be no unexpected or unwelcome consequences... We will have no babies until we want them, no fumbling about putting on French letters or putting in diaphragms. No need to use any messy creams or jellies in the vagina.'

So women were no longer tied down to relying on men for contraception; and whereas previously only men had been able to have intercourse freely with many partners without having to worry, suddenly women felt that they could do the same.

In fact there came about what has been widely known as the 'sexual revolution', which changed the sexual role of women and especially changed their choices about love-making. Until 100 percent effective contraception for women came about, men had in the main been the hunters and women the hunted, in sexual encounters. Now the sexes had become equal and women were just as free as their partners to go looking for sex.

Then came a backlash. Some women who had taken large-dose pills developed blocked arteries or veins – so-called thrombosis – and a few even died. The media publicized this a great deal so that some women were scared and stopped taking the pill without consulting their doctor; and many who did stop the pill became unwantedly pregnant.

Still, this risk of thrombosis was not a very permanent setback, as all the manufacturers had to do was to make pills containing smaller doses of hormones than the originals. These were found to be perhaps even more effective contraceptives. They certainly caused far fewer upsets like painful breasts, not to mention thrombosis.

Then came the other great advance. Intra-uterine devices (IUDs) were invented, or rather rediscovered: desert dwellers put stones into the wombs of she-camels to act as IUDs many years ago. Dr Ernst Graefenburg, a German gynaecologist, had in the 1930s introduced the use of silver inside the uterus for women wanting contraception. He called his devices Graefenburg rings, since they consisted entirely of metal rings. They became unpopular because the metal tended to snap and bore its way into the walls of the womb, and they had other serious side-effects, some of them even more dangerous. When the plastics industry really got going, however, in the 1960s, it was found that plastic IUDs could be put into the womb *comparatively* safely to stop women becoming pregnant (see pages 59–61).

That, too, was a terrific boon: once the coil or intra-uterine device had been fitted, the woman hardly knew it was there. Doctors enthusiastically prescribed and used it as a 'fit-and-forget' method of birth control. Three-quarters of all women who used the IUD got on with it very well indeed.

But in 1986 there was a sudden new setback in that field too. The American firms that had been making and selling Copper Sevens, the most popular intra-uterine devices not only in the United States but throughout the world, stopped making or marketing IUDs because too many women had sued them, claiming they had become infected as a result of wearing their devices. In fact, most of the women could be proved to have had diseases that were sexually transmitted. But the cost and worry of defending IUDs in the courts was just too much for the manufacturers; they decided it was not worth the effort, and pulled out.

Even so, things did not seem too bad. There was still the low-dose pill and the other methods, such as the diaphragm that had been improved and could still be used, even if it did lessen some of the fun (see pages 52–53).

BECOMING INFECTED

But now there has come a far greater awareness that casual sex, sex with many partners, or even occasional sex with someone who has had many partners, can lead to the risk of acquiring something nasty and unexpected such as a sexually transmitted disease, or even cancer.

Of course, sexually transmitted diseases have been around for a long time. They were formerly called venereal diseases (VD), but the term venereal disease covered only four quite specific illnesses: syphilis and gonorrhoea, and two others which were far less common. Even a big upsurge in STDs in the past was not too serious, because doctors could cure most of them and if they really tried could cure virtually all of them. What is more, they could diagnose an STD very quickly. As a result, syphilis, which a hundred years ago was fatal, has become much less serious and much less frequent, and now it even looks as though it could disappear altogether because of penicillin.

However, recently there appeared two STDs which, try as they may, doctors can as yet find no way of curing. The first of these was herpes (see pages 85–86) which apparently will always recur, even though each attack is less serious than the first and can be cut short by the use of new drugs. But herpes is a bearable illness. It is not nearly as serious as some writers in the popular newspapers have made out, and it hardly ever kills the sufferer, though it can endanger the life of a baby being born through an infected vagina.

Then came a terrible disease.

AIDS (Acquired Immune Deficiency Syndrome) is, like herpes, a disease that is transmitted from one person to another by a virus, but in all other ways it is a totally different form of illness. This really is a killer disease – if you like, a replacement for syphilis.

It took some time before the virus, HIV (see page 72), was identified. But even the identification of the virus has done nothing as yet to make it possible to curtail the course of the disease. There is not yet any vaccine against it, nor any cure once the virus has got into the bloodstream and shown itself by the signs and symptoms of the fully developed AIDS disease. But early diagnosis can help to limit its spread once the person has been warned that he or she is infectious, and if the person has enough conscience and sense of responsibility to avoid passing it on.

One thing is certain, that AIDS is transmitted through the blood via a cut or sore, and so far it is nearly always caught by sexual transmission. As will be stressed elsewhere in this book, unless two people have a very long-standing relationship and know that there have been no other partners on either side, intercourse or fellatio (see pages 33–38 and 40) should only take place with the protection of a condom against the risk of infection. No one who takes drugs intravenously should ever share a needle though this is becoming one of the key ways by which the virus is introduced into the heterosexual population. But there is no need to worry about the fork or glass in the restaurant, the sneezing waitress or the person leaning against you in the tube. The only exceptions to this usual manner of transmission have been people like haemophiliacs, who need injected blood products to make their own blood able to clot and to cease bleeding, and people in need of blood transfusions; but now there are safeguards to detect and prevent AIDS transmission in this way (see page 75).

The sexual revolution: has it been a success?
It is quite clear that the present generation of young people is liberated in a way that previous generations never were. In the older days, fear of pregnancy put a very strong brake on 'going all the way'. So did the fear of catching VD.

In the heady days of the 1960s and early 1970s, the invention of good contraception like the low-dose pill and the plastic devices made for easy, carefree intercourse, and this was seized upon by girls perhaps even more than by boys. There seemed no limit to the amount of sexual experience one could have before marriage, or even after marriage, because it was all harmless. Pregnancies were not likely to occur. If they did, terminations were easily obtained. Diseases were not likely to be caught. If they were, they could be cured quite easily. There were doctors willing and able to help out those with STDs, or girls with unwanted pregnancies. That is why free-for-all sex with pleasure all round for everybody seemed so attractive to so many.

The worry about AIDS and herpes has put a very big cloud over the sexual scene, and changed people's behaviour. So what is sexual liberation today? How, in fact, do people behave in the second half of the 1980s?

When I asked a group of young women whether they thought many of them were likely to have several partners before marriage and if so, how many, they all said that unless one was brought up very strictly, for instance in an Asian community with strict parental supervision, or in a Greek Orthodox community where religious beliefs are overwhelmingly in favour of virginity until marriage, girls do have a lot of partners before marriage. The group I spoke to included one or two Irish Catholic nurses, who were surprisingly forthcoming in what they had to say.

They all agreed that it was normal to have several partners before marriage. One of them told me she thought the average would be about three, but then gradually the numbers rose until another, recently married, said she thought somewhere between 15 and 30 was much more likely to be the number, if a girl didn't marry before she was 30. Heterosexual men tend to have more partners than women, say about half as many again; but homosexuals have at least two or three times as many partners in a year, and for many of them this pattern continues if they form no long-term relationship. These girls knew very well that I would not moralize or sit in judgement. I believe doctors cannot really help people if they do not understand

what is going on around them, or if they think they can change
or have a duty to change the behaviour of society by moralizing
to individuals. They cannot and do not, and they become
useless to their patients if they are no longer sympathetic and
understanding about the motives which drive people to behave
sexually in the way they do.

What do people do, and why?

The most common behaviour is to have a heterosexual
relationship ('hetero' is a Greek word meaning 'other', i.e. not
the same). So this means relationships between boys and girls
and men and women, occasionally between older men and
younger girls, and rather less frequently between older women
and younger men. The word homosexual does not come from
the Latin word 'homo', a man, but from the Greek word
'homos', meaning 'the same'. So someone who has sex with a
partner of the same sex is known as a homosexual. The word
lesbian, meaning a homosexual woman, comes from the name
of the Greek island, Lesbos, where the sixth-century poetess
Sappho, who was homosexual, lived. Sapphic means the same
as lesbian.

Why do people have sex? That seems like a silly question.
Everybody knows that sex is a great urge like hunger, thirst and
the need to laugh. But there is no need to have a lot of partners
to enjoy sex. One reason why so many people do have so many
partners is that they find sex is *not* always all that enjoyable, so
they hurry on to find satisfaction elsewhere. Another reason is
just the opposite. Sex is *so* enjoyable that they want to try it
with others. For them, each new contact is an adventure, and
adventure can be elating. Each new partner is a conquest, and
conquest can be exciting and morale-boosting. Many people of
both sexes simply crave excitement.

A lot of it is done for 'kicks'. The very young get a kick out of
doing something that makes them feel independent of their
parents, or, if they come from a split home, independent of the
parent with whom they live. Many young people are
antagonistic towards their parents. Many others just want to
escape from a perhaps small and confined home: surely life has
more to offer than that restricted environment, and surely

meeting the opposite sex, something parents often regard with caution, is going to be a great thrill?

It seems fine to go disco-dancing and pick up someone for sex. The opportunities are almost unrestricted. Parents may be out at work or out enjoying themselves, so the young people could be uninterrupted in one of their homes. If not, there is the odd corner behind the disco, in the back of the car, or a place in the park, or a field near the village.

There are a lot of parents, too, who encourage girls to have lovers. A surprising number, knowing that their daughters are very likely to have sex relations with boys and worried that they may come home with an unwelcome pregnancy, encourage them to use effective birth control and even take them to the doctor. No liberal-minded GP, gynaecologist or birth control specialist practises for long without being approached by a mother for advice about her young daughter's contraception needs.

Mrs Victoria Gillick, who started the long-running famous case when she said she wanted to be sure that no doctor would give her young daughters birth control advice without her knowledge and consent, was completely out of touch with reality. She did not realize that there is a 'swinging' generation of parents who take exactly the opposite view. She did not realize either how many parents turn a blind eye, when really they know that their daughters are involved in sexual relationships.

Unfortunately, very few parents give their sons and daughters enough information about the importance of the condom, both as a contraceptive measure and as a protection against infection, and very few try to instil in them a sense of sexual or moral responsibility.

BEING HURT EMOTIONALLY

Yes, it may be quite good fun, but in so many relationships there is something sought and not found, something more than excitement or flattery wanted, and so another attempt is made with a different partner.

People never think about how they will feel when a relationship breaks against their wish, as it may well do, and as it must do if there are many partners. They do not worry about emotional hurt, particularly if every brief relationship is enjoyable but not serious: then there is, in fact, very little chance of emotional damage, particularly if no infection has been caught and no pregnancy risked. If the sex has been good, that's fine, and if it has not – good riddance to that partner. Both boys and girls do get over a break in a short relationship easily, but it is certainly not so easy when the relationship has lasted longer, or seems to have settled down into something pretty stable and permanent. If then one partner wants to break away for a relationship with another person, the partner left behind is going to be hurt, and sometimes very hurt indeed. That is why they seek love and reassurance time and time again.

Many girls and boys feel that 'sex' is a thing to try, that losing virginity is a 'step' that has to be taken. Many 14- or 15-year-old girls unfortunately feel left out of things if they have not had a boy make love to them completely, and that they must be abnormal if it hasn't happened by the time they are seventeen or eighteen. Too many girls have intercourse not because they really want to, but because they fear that otherwise they will not be in with the in-crowd. When relationships are built on this flimsy ground they are almost bound to collapse, and very often the girl cannot then turn to her parents, if they have been unaware of her relationships, or antagonistic towards them. It can be worse still if the parents have encouraged that particular relationship: she will feel a failure and rejected by them as well as by her partner. The same is largely true of boys too. So the only person a young man or woman feels he or she can turn to is another partner. A relationship started for the wrong reasons leads to further disappointment and to more promiscuity, and the longer it goes on and the more partners there are, the less likely anyone is to find what he or she really needs.

When I asked one girl whether she had lots of partners she said, 'No. I am not really promiscuous.' When I pressed her she admitted she had had 100 partners in less than a year and had not fully enjoyed the relationship with any one of them! And when pressed still further as to why she did it, she admitted that she just wanted to feel wanted. Some doctors, even those filled with sympathy, feel that this wasteful, frantic chase is a 'rubbishing' of one's own personality, leaving a person with less and less self-esteem. The search may go on and on and become more and more desperate as hopes decrease, so that the victim ends up thinking 'It's just me.' It is not. But one has to give things a real chance. Relationships take time to develop into affection, and affection is what matters in sexual relationships. One of my patients was a prostitute for years and was terribly surprised when one of her clients fell in love with her desperately and deeply. They have been married some years now and it is a very happy marriage.

One of the most painful effects of 'rubbishing' that can result from a long series of short-term promiscuous relationships, especially if there has been an infection along the way, is a feeling of guilt or of being worthless or, even worse, of being dirty. People can end up, particularly if they come from a strictly religious family, thinking 'Perhaps my parents are right – God is punishing me.' But it is not like that. There is always the possibility of a strong, warm relationship. It is nice to be wanted and to be fancied, and to want and to fancy, and in the end there is nearly always a partner who will respect you and love you for what you are.

In life there are happy kids and unhappy kids, frightened and confident kids, but the pressures on the unhappy and on the frightened can be very heavy indeed.

So many young people, particularly from broken homes, consciously or not may seek revenge against the parent they feel has broken up what should have been a stable home and hurt the other parent. They do not understand that both members of a couple nearly always generate arguments equally. Some other young adults, of course, rebel against both parents. These people are hurt again if they are then rejected cruelly or carelessly by the partner they have chosen, particularly if they thought their own partnership would last.

At the outset of a love affair a good sexual experience will help to establish the emotional side of the relationship, which takes much longer to develop. It is a big step to move into a home together and an even bigger step to marry. However, although the emotional and friendship side of a marriage is very important indeed, and the sex life less so, when love-making does go badly wrong it can wreck a marriage, particularly if sex was good beforehand.

There may be sexual difficulties when babies come along, but that is part of the learning process a couple must share, because women have instilled into them that their role in life is that of a mother and now that they have fulfilled that role, for a short time at least they are sexually fulfilled. Many couples come for medical advice because sex has become less good after the birth of a baby. With patience things will improve, but not if the man, disappointed, thinks his wife no longer cares for him and dashes off to find consolation in another partner's arms. The arms will often be waiting but the consolation will be empty.

So, in order not to be hurt by that apparent rejection and the resulting betrayal, people should realize that having a baby is a very big step indeed, and no pregnancy should be started without being certain that a child is wanted. Terminations are not the answer. No woman gets over a termination completely, even if she says she has, until she has another baby in her arms to replace the one that was lost. This may not be for many years, and if it never comes the disappointment may last for ever. Today there is effective contraception, so therefore there is a choice as to whether to have a baby or not; the decision should be made consciously and should not be left to chance.

Even worse than love-making going wrong is the discovery that one has been infected by a trusted partner: that gives rise to a sense of betrayal. It has to be admitted, however, that many young people have in the past considered a sexually transmitted disease as an incidental happening in their sex lives, nothing to get worked up about. Obviously they are *not* going to think that now, if they have a mortally dangerous disease like AIDS.

When the one who has been infected realizes his or her own lover has been the cause of infection, it is very difficult for the relationship to continue, because it *is* a betrayal, both emotionally and physically, particularly if the infection has been transmitted recklessly in an 'I couldn't care less' attitude. Many times, however, the person doing the infecting is completely ignorant of the presence of a disease and is shocked when he or she understands what has been done and, perhaps, what has been lost.

This book has been written to try and show the way to avoid the physical and emotional damage that results from failure to avoid pregnancy, failure to avoid infectious disease and failure to avoid unnecessary emotional hurt. It is possible to avoid unsafe sex. It is very possible and not too difficult to have safe, enjoyable and very rewarding sex.

2
WHAT IS SEX?

The word 'sex' originally meant those characteristics, that made a man or a woman clearly male or female. It is also used as an adjective, as in sex education, sexual transmission, sex hygiene, sexual gratification and sexual discrimination. It has now become an abbreviation for sexual intercourse, but it also includes those feelings or behaviours that come about because of the need to satisfy the sexual instinct. This need is as important for the continuation of the human race as keeping fed, keeping warm and keeping alive.

Sexual pleasure can be obtained without full sexual intercourse and even without a partner, providing some sexual fantasy is aroused.

Both men and women masturbate by themselves to obtain relief of sexual tension and to satisfy something in the sexual urge. Couples do mutually masturbate one another, and may obtain as much sexual satisfaction from that as from full intercourse. Lesbian women, of course, cannot have full bodily sexual connection with one another in the same way as couples of the opposite sex do, and as male homosexuals may, so mutual masturbation or using a dildo (see page 41) are their most frequent forms of sexual relief.

EROGENOUS ZONES

Another important way to give sexual satisfaction is to stimulate the erogenous zones of the body. An erogenous zone is a part of the body that is sexually sensitive: stroking, touching or kissing there will result in sexual pleasure for both partners, and maybe in a heightened desire for intercourse.

Stimulating erogenous zones causes sensations to go up the

nerves from the skin through the spinal column to the brain, where they are recognized either as something pleasant or unpleasant. For instance, for some people it is erogenous to smell a perfume but smelling bad breath is usually the exact opposite. So, the inside of the nose is an erogenous zone for the stimulus of smell – a different kind of erogenous turning-on. There is hardly any part of the body that is not for someone an erogenous zone. I was quite startled to find deep love bites on the lowest part of the neck just above the right shoulder of one of my patients. She explained that being bitten there (but not on the left side!) was for her the most sexually stimulating thing, and that she could invariably obtain an orgasm if her partner bit her there, so long as he did not really hurt her.

There is nothing so strange and unexpected as to learn what acts as a 'turn-on' for some people and a 'turn-off' for others. But for most people just seeing one's partner stripping naked, and stroking and being stroked over areas of the skin and the genital organs are what really act as sexual stimulation.

The whole surface of the skin can, in theory, when touched in certain ways, stimulate erotic thoughts and reactions, but this is only *potentially*. The mood and the setting have to be right, as well as the partners being right for one another. Men tend to like squeezing women's buttocks and some women may enjoy this. No woman really likes having her bottom pinched, which too many men seem to think is enjoyable for women at any time. There are many women who really dislike having certain parts of their bodies touched at all, and that, too, varies from woman to woman. It is obvious that if a girl is very ticklish she is not going to be stimulated sexually by a partner lightly rubbing the soles of her feet or under her armpits, but she may be very much stimulated if gentle movements are made by her partner's fingers creeping gradually up the insides of her legs. Similarly, most women like to have their breasts touched but not in such a way that they are tickled, nor so heavily that the breasts are bruised. Sometimes, however, particularly during the week before a period is due, breasts are so tender that women do not like to have them touched at all.

For many men, kissing his partner's nipples is sexually stimulating for him; but not all women want this, although very many do. So, if sexual stimuation is going to be carried on so intensely as to bring on an orgasm or an ejaculation as a substitute for full intercourse, each partner has to get to know what the other really likes and wants; and neither should be offended or sensitive if the other tells him or her what to do. Men still tend to be stupidly conceited in thinking that they know all about how to make love. When they change partners they cannot possibly know what that particular new partner really wants unless they ask and are told, or unless both are happy to find out by experiment.

One does not necessarily have to touch or be touched for sexual stimulation. Everybody has his or her own odour, and for some the mere characteristic smell of the partner's body is sexually stimulating. It may be a scent or cologne that is exciting, which is why perfumes sell so well. Blind people can certainly have completely full sex lives, but most couples do rely also at some stage in their love-making on sight as well as touch and smell and sound; the expression in the partner's eyes can be all-important. In parks, cafés and restaurants couples hold hands and do apparently nothing except look lovingly in one another's eyes; and one knows that this is often a preliminary to more intimate contact when they leave.

Many people like to have the backs of their ears stroked gently, or the lobes of their ears fondled, and also like the back of the neck to be rubbed smoothly. Kissing, of course, can be a big stimulus, as well as French kissing – putting the tongue in the partner's mouth; the inside and the roof of the mouth, therefore, as well as the tongue, may be erogenous zones.

If full intercourse is to be avoided, either to minimize the risks of pregnancy or the transmission of disease, and yet pleasure still to be given and received, people should realize that their partner may be unpredictable yet still responsive, and that each individual is totally different in the way he or she reacts to being touched sexually in one or other part of the body. Hardly anyone likes having the same things done each time in the same order in a mechanical sort of way, because that is boring and too predictable and is therefore sexually not exciting. It is also artistically bad sexual behaviour, rather like serving up the same dish at every meal; good sexual behaviour can be and should be an art which both partners should share in.

People who are ignorant of the erogenous zones and their importance in a happy sex life cannot achieve as fully satisfying love lives as can those who know something about their own anatomy and the anatomy of the opposite sex. So it is essential to understand something about the structure of the sex organs.

FEMALE EXTERNAL SEXUAL ORGANS AS EROGENOUS ZONES

Men tend to know much more than women about their own sexual anatomy because most of the male sexual organs are easily visible.

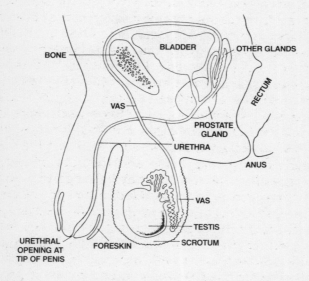

The major part of women's sex organs are internal, and even the external organs are visible only if a women has both the curiosity and the necessary desire to look at herself with a mirror. However, even that is not easy, because the outside lips of the vulva, the labia majora, have to be separated with two fingers and usually that is better done with the fingers of both hands. The mirror then has somehow to be balanced and the woman's neck bent forward, all of which demands some acrobatic skill! (Labia is the plural of the Latin word for lip. The inside lips are called the labia minora and extend from the clitoris towards the back passage.)

I am constantly surprised at how little women know about their own bodies. For instance, very few know that the outside hole of the water pipe, the urethra, through which urine is passed from the bladder, is near but not at the very front of what is called the vestibule or entrance to the vagina. The clitoris is at least an inch in front again of the urethra. Women do not pass urine through the clitoris as men do through the penis.

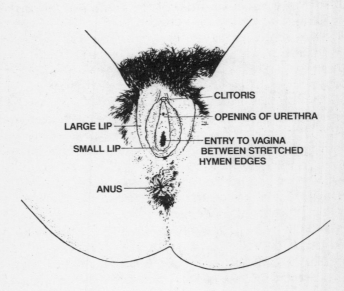

LARGE LIP

SMALL LIP

ANUS

CLITORIS

OPENING OF URETHRA

ENTRY TO VAGINA
BETWEEN STRETCHED
HYMEN EDGES

Also, too few women realize that orgasm is a thing that has to be learned. Very, very few early sexual relationships end in orgasm for the woman. It is something for which there has to be a learning process – preferably with the same stable partner. Seeking for it without the willingness to learn gradually will lead to disappointment.

The clitoris

The clitoris is the most highly developed of all the erogenous zones in the human body. It is covered by a hood or prepuce just like the foreskin of the uncircumcized penis, and, like the penis, it is fixed to the front of the bones that make the pelvis. It is only in these ways that the two correspond. The clitoris is *not* a small penis, because its function is different, although both most certainly are sexual organs. The clitoris is much smaller than the penis, but millimetre for millimetre it is much more intensively endowed with nerves that pick up sensations. Its sole function is for sexual stimulation. The penis, of course, is used for passing urine or for ejaculating semen; it cannot perform both functions at the same time, nor can a man pass urine easily when he has an erection.

It is only relatively recently, within the last 20 years or so, that doctors themselves have found out much about the behaviour of the clitoris in sexual excitement. Clitorises, like noses, come in different shapes and sizes, the only thing being absolutely consistent is that the organ is very rarely indeed much more than half an inch across; more usually it may be as small as a tenth of an inch across. It receives sensations, say, from the partner's fingers touching it, and it transforms the sensations into a sexual stimulus. However, the clitoris can change its shape and size if another part of the body is being stimulated, for instance the breasts, but not if they are being stimulated by a baby breast-feeding. Often, if the breast is being sucked by a man to please himself, it may have no effect on his partner's clitoris. Masters and Johnson in their book [Human Sexual Response (J. and A. Churchill Ltd), 1966] point out that the shaft of the clitoris may be quite long and thin and surmounted by a small tip or glans, or it may be short and thick and have a larger tip. They were unable to measure its size accurately either at rest or when being stimulated sexually.

It is not possible to tell by looking at a clitoris how it will react to stimulation, because every woman is different and every stimulus is different. A woman may be stimulated either by touching the clitoris, or by rubbing the whole of the mons, which is the fatty area in front of it, or by holding over it the two lips at either side. She may also be stimulated by having some other erogenous zone touched or even by a sexual fantasy such as looking at a video, although visual aids as a rule do not turn women on as they do men.

The clitoris nearly always responds, in the woman who is keen to go further with that particular partner, by the glans at the tip enlarging, so that the hood above it becomes tightly stretched, giving rise to increasing sexual tension.

Once the glans at the tip has become larger, the diameter of the shaft increases, but there is no erection like that of the penis. At the same time usually the labia minora also begin to swell up to at least twice their normal size. If the shaft of the clitoris gets longer, which it does in only a small percentage of women when it is being stimulated directly (but always does if the woman is going to go on to orgasm) the body of the clitoris seems to retreat towards the vagina, up against the bone in front of the pelvis. It is as though the prepuce comes forward to protect the glans from being too strongly stimulated. And, disappointingly for a woman who is being stimulated by her partner's tongue (see pages 38–40) the clitoris seems to go away from the tongue, and she may accuse her partner of losing contact. It is not the partner's fault at all, because the clitoris itself has, as it were, doubled back; but if as a result sexual stimulation diminishes, down comes the clitoris again and presents itself for further stimulation.

By that time, however, usually the lips of the vulva have become so engorged that they take over as the sexually responsive organs, or, if the penis has been introduced, as it often has with intercourse at this stage, the shaft of the penis itself, providing the couple are in a good position, may stimulate a clitoris that has retracted.

This rather full description of the clitoris and its behaviour has been given because clitoris stimulation is perhaps the most important part of getting women sexually excited, although many people are completely unaware of this and girls are often too shy to explain, even in this liberated and enlightened age. Many, many women can even achieve orgasm just from gentle stimulation of the clitoris by fingers, or by stimulation with the partner's tongue, or indirectly by stimulation of the breasts, without full intercourse being needed.

Of course, most women feel that they have not 'given themselves' properly if they have not agreed to intercourse by the penis being inserted into the vagina. Many women, certainly, want above all to be penetrated just as men want to do the penetrating. But this does not mean that penetration is always necessary for a woman to be carried a long way towards sexual satisfaction, or having an orgasm.

Penetration is a totally different matter from external stimulation. Although Masters and Johnson say there is no chance of orgasm just from sensations felt deep inside the vagina, their conclusions are probably not true. The vaginal walls themselves may well be erogenous zones and even more so the cervix (the neck of the womb). Recently people have been talking about the front wall of the vagina, the so-called G-spot, being an erogenous zone, and there are many women who say they do not get a proper orgasm without something penetrating the vagina and going right up to the top of it where the cervix is.

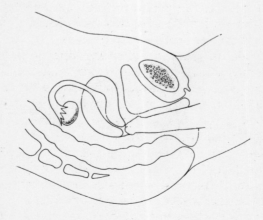

MALE EROGENOUS ZONES

These are not very different in position from the female ones. Men also like to be kissed. Men also like to have their ears stroked gently, and their necks touched. They like to have arms encircle them and to feel lips against theirs and against their faces and bodies. They like to have the skin on their arms and the insides of their legs gently stroked. They like to have their backs rubbed and even sometimes to have the spine massaged quite vigorously. Men often like to have the top of the penis kissed or sucked; this can be immensely stimulating sexually. Above all, they like to have their penises gently stroked, responding better and more strongly to having the under surface stroked than the top surface. Men also like to have the scrotum, in which their testes (their balls) are situated, very gently handled. They certainly do not like to have it squeezed. That hurts, and is a turn-off instead of a turn-on.

With relaxed, slow intercourse, experienced couples will find a variety of different 'spots' and positions to be erogenous for them.

3
HOW DO PEOPLE HAVE SEX? IS IT SAFE?

There is an enormous variety of sexual activity. Sexual response starts very young indeed: it starts in the cradle and can continue to the grave. Obviously sexual activity will vary at different ages, both in kind and in intensity.

KISSING

This is the most common preliminary step in love-making. It not only acts as a powerful sexual stimulant but also as a demonstration of affection and love. Some couples will kiss for ages and do no more than that. Body kisses are certainly sexually very stimulating, but of course not all kissing is sexual. Women who are by no means lesbian kiss one another when they meet, and it is normal practice for friends of the opposite sex to kiss one another without any intention of there being any further sexual contact at all. In many countries it is accepted practice that men, too, will kiss each other on both cheeks when they meet. In these instances it is no more than a form of greeting. But continued kissing for a long period of time is certainly sexual, whether it is between partners of the opposite sex or the same sex when they want to stimulate one another.

Planting kisses all over the body is an affectionate sexual activity, and in its own way shows how one partner admires and respects the whole of the other's body. Love bites are an extreme form of kissing, but they should never be so firm as to draw blood.

Is it *safe*?

Yes, relatively so. But if either partner has a sore on the mouth or tongue, or has herpes spots (see page 85) it is obviously unsafe, because germs in an infected sore on the lips, or in the mouth or on the tongue can be transmitted by kissing and especially by French kissing.

However, sores in the mouth are seldom unfelt or unseen, so infections there are more obvious than those inside the vagina, or penis or bladder. Although it is possible to catch infections from kissing, relatively few are caught that way.

'Social' kissing is always safe.

MASTURBATION

Masturbation does not necessarily end in orgasm. Little boys and little girls in their cots can be seen playing with their sexual organs – their own, that is, not one another's!

Boys usually start this when they are about six or seven months old, or maybe a little earlier, and girls usually by the time they are a year old. All the boys do is to touch their penises, and although it is possible for boys to have an erection when they are only a few days old, as a result of hormones from their mothers circulating in their blood, they do not often obtain erections from touching themselves at this very young age. Still, it is obviously enjoyable because you can see them gurgling away in their prams, clearly getting a lot of pleasure from fondling the penis and even the scrotum. Boys do not rub their penises until later, usually by the age of about two or so. Some, at the ages of three, four and five years or so, will touch their penises even through their trousers. They would not do it if they did not like it.

Some doctors have thought that sucking thumbs was an alternative to masturbation, but this seems doubtful. Thumb-sucking is probably a form of self-comfort more than a form of sexual activity, whereas playing with the penis must provide some sexual sensation.

Very young girls tend not to rub the vulva or the clitoris so much as to press their thighs together, to rock to and fro against a pillow or even against a doll held near the vulva. They will also clutch at their parents with their legs wide apart and quite clearly lean the vulva against the arm or neck of a person carrying them. It is perfectly normal behaviour.

Some people believe that very young boys and girls do masturbate to the point of having an orgasm, but it is very difficult to show that this is really true, especially as little boys do not ejaculate as older ones do: no semen comes out until the age of puberty or even a little later. Small boys do, however, sometimes have erections when playing with other children. It is quite usual for very young boys and girls to show each other their sexual organs and to satisfy one another's curiosity. I once saw this happen in one of London's smartest restaurants at tea-time, where the parents, unaware, were eating cucumber sandwiches and drinking tea very genteelly while the children were pulling their shorts and knickers aside so that they could look at one another's bodies.

Too many parents try to stop little boys and girls playing with themselves 'down there', telling their children it is a 'dirty thing to do'. Of course it is not 'dirty', and this kind of repression of what the child does instinctively may make him or her associate the idea of sex with dirt or with dirty behaviour, and may in some way blight a boy's or girl's ability to look forward to sex as something wonderful and enjoyable, and, as it should be, tremendously rewarding.

Masturbation to orgasm or ejaculation of semen is very common indeed from the age of about fifteen or sixteen onwards and quite often as young as twelve. Whether this involves feeling guilty or not about it depends entirely on the attitude of parents. Religions have for so long taught that masturbation is something that is frowned upon or bears some penalty, or even that is sinful, that it has become difficult to eradicate these ideas. It used to be taught in English schools that a boy who masturbated could not keep his eye in for sports! Nonsense!

Masturbation stimulated by erotic material is very common indeed and one of the reasons for the sale of sexy videos and 'girlie' magazines, as well as erotic books. Men read these books and masturbate, fantasizing that they are in the situation of the man in the book. Women tend not to be so stimulated by erotic material, at least not to the extent of having an orgasm, but many women do enjoy seeing erotic things. However, equally many are put off by erotic material: magazines showing full-frontal views of men do not have nearly as great a sale as those that show erotic pictures of girls.

Girls masturbate probably almost universally, even if it is not considered ladylike. They do not usually masturbate inside the vagina but by stimulation of the clitoris, and this is more likely to be done by rubbing the lips of the vulva together or manipulating the front of the vulva rather than by touching the clitoris itself, although, of course, that is also done. It is only later, usually after a girl has experienced intercourse, that she may resort to stimulating herself inside the vagina, either by using her fingers or some artificial 'aid', like a dildo, and shaped like a penis. Increasingly, women are using vibrators as an aid to masturbation (see page 41), and some use one on the clitoris to get extra stimulation if they cannot be stimulated with the penis in the vagina during intercourse.

Is it *safe*?

Absolutely. There is nothing unsafe about masturbation for boys or girls or men or women, even if it progresses to ejaculation in men and orgasm in women. It is frowned on by some religions but there is nothing about it that will damage health, and certainly there is no way for anyone to infect themselves by it.

Mutual masturbation is a very common way of obtaining sexual stimulation and satisfaction. Mostly when heterosexual couples mutually masturbate one another to orgasm and ejaculation they do so without intending full sexual intercourse to follow. This is sometimes called heavy petting and very many young people start sexual experience in this way. It probably is the most common form of sexual stimulation short of intercourse.

Is it *safe*?

Yes, it is certainly safer than intercourse from the point of view of not transmitting infection, but care has to be taken to make sure that if the man ejaculates he does not do so too near the woman's vulva, because if semen is spilt on the vulva at about the time the woman is ovulating, the semen, which has movement of its own, can enter the vagina and make her pregnant. By and large, since no great expectations are aroused by this form of sexual behaviour, neither of the couple gets very upset if full sexual satisfaction is not obtained, and therefore there is little emotional damage even if it does not 'work'. Certainly with a little care there is only a very small risk of infection or of pregnancy, but the risk of infection is slightly raised if there is any scratch or cut on the vulva. However, since the AIDS virus, HIV, does take several weeks and even months to show up in a blood test, particular care should be taken to avoid fellatio (see page 40) without using a sheath.

EROTIC DREAMS

Both men and women have erotic dreams. Boys, when they are reaching adolescence, may well not remember the dream which has resulted in emission of semen during the night. Most 'wet dreams' happen just before waking so they wake up having ejaculated and possibly having stained the nightclothes or bedclothes. This may be unfortunate, but it is inevitable and certainly nothing of which to be ashamed, but boys do sometimes get upset by wet dreams if they have not been warned that these are likely to occur.

Girls do not have orgasm from dreams when they are deeply asleep. But they certainly do touch themselves in a half-awake state either just before going to sleep or on waking up. They may even, without being completely conscious of the fact, masturbate in their sleep to orgasm.

It is *safe*?

Certainly. Erotic dreams are an absolutely normal stage of sexual development and also happen to mature men and women who are used to an active sex life, if they are temporarily deprived of it by the absence of their partners. It is a completely healthy thing to happen.

HETEROSEXUAL INTERCOURSE

The title of this book is *Safe Sex*, so it is not about how to avoid sex but about how to avoid unsafe sex. Intercourse without contraception between a couple who have no infections whatsoever, who love one another and desire one another and understand how to fulfil one another, constitutes the most sublime of all experiences. However, unless the couple have a very long-standing relationship and know that there have been no other partners on either side, intercourse should only take place with the protection of a condom against the risk of infection.

There are books that describe in great detail the different positions and variations adopted in intercourse. All that will be done here is to describe briefly the positions heterosexuals most frequently use.

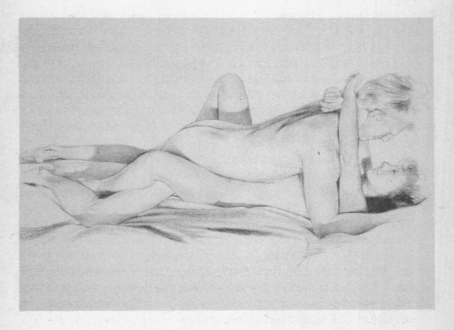

1 The missionary position, in which the woman, lying on her back with her legs spread open and her knees bent, is penetrated through her vulva into her vagina. In this position she cannot make quite as strong movements as the man, but it is the most frequently used position for satisfactory intercourse. Orgasm for the woman will come with practice.

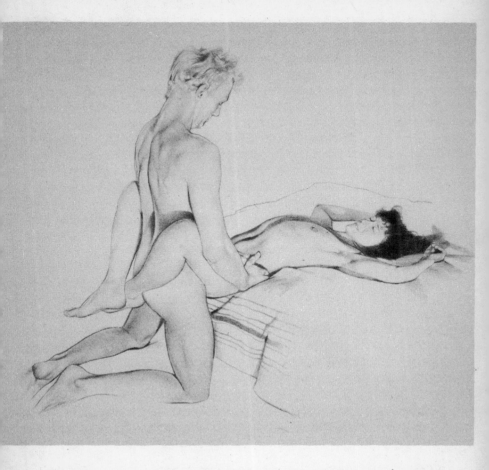

2   The woman lies on a bed or even the edge of a table with her buttocks just over the edge, and the man either kneels or stands beside her and inserts his penis in that way. It is just a variation of the first position and certainly makes a change.

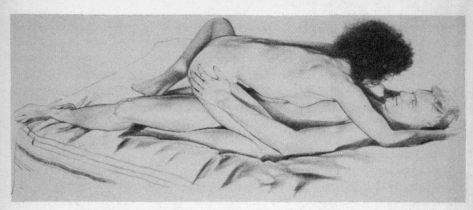

3 The man lies on the bed and the woman squats over his erect penis.

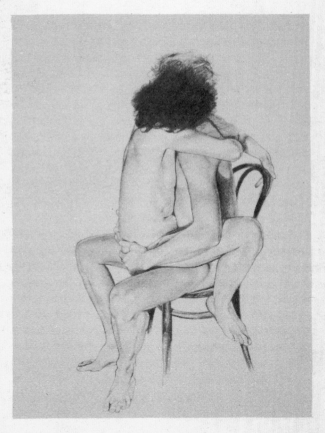

4 (Opposite, below) Both in sitting positions, the man usually on a chair and the woman lowering herself on to his penis, either facing him or facing away.

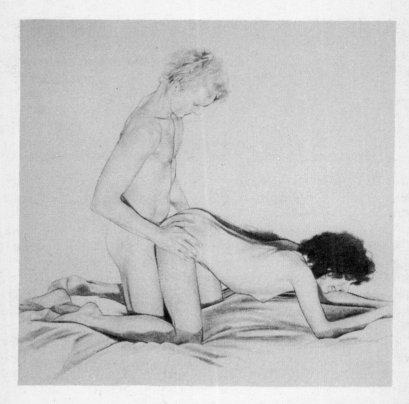

5 Rear entry vaginal intercourse, in which the woman lies on her knees and elbows or on her side with her knees drawn up and the man enters her vagina from behind. There is quite close body contact this way and it makes a good variation. Alternatively, rear entry can be effected with the woman leaning over the back of a chair with her legs apart (see that the chair is strong enough not to topple over!) and the man standing behind her enters her vagina that way.

(For more information about intercourse, see Further Reading, page 111.)

Are these *safe*?

Normally, yes, all except the rear entry position, when sometimes the woman's bladder may be bruised, giving rise to attacks of cystitis (see pages 81–82). But if intercourse is not meant to result in pregnancy and if birth control is not used, there is a very strong risk of every act of intercourse ending in a pregnancy.

And if either party has a sexually transmissible disease, such forms of intercourse are *the* way to transmit it, so it can then be very unsafe indeed, in any position.

ORO-GENITAL SEX

This form of sexual activity involves mouth contact with the sex organs of the partner. Again, unless two people have a long-standing and exclusive sexual relationship, it is wise to have the protection of a condom against the risk of infection.

Oro-genital sex is certainly not a perversion and for many it is a highly refined form of love-making. It goes without saying, however, that germs can be passed to a partner whether by kissing on the mouth, on the genitalia, or elsewhere, because they can enter the body anywhere where the skin is cut, or thin or different, as it is in the mouth and the vagina.

Although the genital organs should always be kept clean by washing, 'fresheners', bubble baths, scents and deodorants are more likely to give rise to skin rashes than to be sexually attractive, so they should be avoided. It is best to wash the genitalia with soap and water before love-making.

Cunnilingus

This means the man uses his lips and his tongue to stimulate part of the woman's vulva, in particular the clitoris, by sucking, kissing and by tongue movements. The name cunnilingus comes from the Latin words for the external female genital organs and for the tongue. In everyday language it is known as 'eating pussy' and doubtless many other phrases are used too.

Cunnilingus is enjoyed by millions of couples, including lesbians, of course. There used to be a hang-up about it, left over from the Victorian attitude that sexual organs must be something dirty, and that therefore while it was all right to touch them with fingers and with the sexual organs of the opposite sex, kissing them was not a clean thing to do. Now, oro-genital sex is almost universally practised by younger people, either as a preliminary to full sexual intercourse or as a substitute for it. Men like doing it and women like having it done to them. There is, as in every other form of sexual activity, a need to learn the skill of how to do it most effectively, but having the clitoris kissed and licked with the right kind of tongue movements can be one of the most sexually stimulating experiences for the woman. It is comparatively easy to excite a woman in this way up to orgasm, because the tongue, unlike the fingers, is not nearly so likely to bruise the clitoris or to press too hard and cause pain.

The genital organs have a particular odour, especially on sexual excitement, and while for some partners this is provocative, for others it is off-putting and makes them unable or unwilling to have oral sex.

Many also still baulk at genital kissing because the genitalia serve the double purpose of sex and of passing urine. Stale urine is smelly and 'dirty', and so by implication the hole through which it is passed must be too. But fresh urine is not dirty: it is a sterile fluid which usually only becomes infected when germs in the air get to it. So neither is the hole through which urine is passed dirty. It is, furthermore, easy to wash after passing urine to make doubly sure of cleanliness. So kissing the sex organs, as well as stroking with the tongue and even sucking, can be practised without fear of contamination or of becoming dirty.

Is it *safe*?

Well, no girl ever became pregnant from being kissed; and if it is used as a substitute for full intercourse it is certainly an absolutely safe way of avoiding pregnancy.

On the other hand, a partner can be infected with gonorrhoea in the mouth, although that is extremely unlikely. But it is possible, if the woman has a syphilis sore on her vulva, for that to be transferred to the man's lips. Equally, if the man has a sore in his mouth, he can transfer it to the woman. The one infection that is very easily transferred by either partner in this way is herpes.

Fellatio

Kissing, licking and sucking the penis is known technically as fellatio, or, more commonly, either as 'giving head' or 'going down'. The name comes from the Latin word for sucking.

A woman can, if she keeps her lips tightly rounded, imitate for the man the sensation of the penis going through the vulva, and if she makes repeated massaging movements with her lips up and down the penis she can drive a man frantic. It is certainly possible to excite a boy or man sufficiently to make him reach orgasm this way, but it is probably used more as foreplay.

The idea of letting a man ejaculate into her mouth is unacceptable to large numbers of women, but if he withdraws from the mouth just before he is going to ejaculate she can then, by masturbating his penis with her moistened hand, allow him to ejaculate outside her. This does not lessen the risks of her catching an infection from the penis, which will be avoided only if the man wears a sheath. Condoms do, of course, diminish sexual excitement for both, and the taste of the rubber may be physically revolting to the partner who is doing the sucking. The imaginative manufacturers of sexual aids have now come up with condoms with different flavours.

In the position known as the '69 position', the couple lie facing one another but with each partner's head pointing towards the other one's feet. In theory, at any rate, it is possible for cunnilingus and fellatio to be carried on at the same time and even for both to reach a climax simultaneously. It is not as easy as it may sound.

Is it *safe*?

The risks of acquiring infection from fellatio, especially if a condom is worn, are low. In the gay community fellatio is now more commonly practised than it was before the advent of AIDS; it may even become more commonly practised than anal intercourse, since the risks are so much less. However, fellatio is frowned upon by some proportion of the gay community.

SEXUAL AIDS

There are sex shops in all large cities and even in some small towns. One of the things they sell, apart from frilly underwear, unusual forms of condoms and erotic pictures, are sexual aids. These have as their purpose either to be a substitute for a partner, or to improve sexual performance.

Vibrators

One of the ways for a woman who wishes to be penetrated to achieve satisfaction but does not allow her boyfriend to wear a sheath, is for her to masturbate him while he inserts a vibrator into her vagina. These vibrators are usually made of plastic, and some are shaped like a penis; they vibrate by the movement of a battery-operated motor. Not all vibrators can be inserted into the vagina; they can also be used to stimulate the clitoris or the penis in foreplay or even during intercourse, or just simply for masturbation.

Dildoes

These are usually made of plastic and are shaped exactly like a penis. They may be used by lesbians, one of whom feels that something should be inserted in the vagina, or they may be used by girls to masturbate themselves.

Are they *safe*?

They are safe to use provided they are not shared. If they are used by anybody else, they must be properly sterilized afterwards before further use. The best way to do this is to wash them in a strong disinfectant or better still, if they can stand it, to boil them. Of course vibrators with batteries inside them cannot be boiled. The answer therefore is, if you do have a sexual aid, keep it personal, as the risk of catching infection from something that has been used by other people, while not as great as of catching it from actual intercourse, is still very real.

HOMOSEXUALITY

Homosexuality is a state of being in which a person is mainly sexually attracted to other people of the same sex. Male homosexuals are now colloquially known as gays and female homosexuals are also known as lesbians. There are lesbian couples who play roles in which the dominant partner, or the partner who takes the more active physical side of the relationship, does dress and behave more like a man than a woman, while the other partner dresses and behaves as any other woman would. But most lesbians cannot be recognized as different from other women.

Homosexuality in a non-sexual sense, by which is meant just preferring the company of the same sex, is normal and natural throughout life. Very young children do not mind whether they play with other children of the same or the opposite sex. From the age of about four or five until puberty, boys tend to prefer to be with boys and play rougher games than girls do; and girls prefer mainly to be with girls. They also tend to look down on members of the opposite sex in those age groups. Later, during and after adolescence, youngsters gradually prefer to be with a member of the opposite sex but of course not exclusively. Many adult men also feel much more at home in male company, for example, in rugger clubs or drinking in a pub. But this does not mean that their sexual inclinations are for members of the same sex, any more than members of women's hockey teams or the Women's Institute are likely to be sexually attracted to other women. All men and women have some homosexuality in their makeup: a very low level of bisexuality (see pages 44–45) is essential, otherwise male friendships could not exist, and nor could female friendships.

Society frequently used to call people who were sexually attracted exclusively to members of the same sex 'perverts'. Doctors thought then that this state, which is so different from the sexual orientation of most people, was determined mainly by the attitudes their parents had towards them when they were children. For instance, a father hoping for a son may perhaps turn his daughter into a tomboy. Alternatively, a mother wishing desperately for a daughter may be disappointed when a boy is born and may, consciously or not, refuse to accept his gender. She may keep him in old-fashioned garments when he should be in rompers or shorts; she may insist on keeping his hair long and curled. She may do everything she can to keep him tied to her apron-strings. Later, when he goes to school, his overly feminine appearance may make other boys consider him a 'sissy'. According to now discredited ideas, this early childhood experience laid the pattern for later homosexuality.

It is now accepted that this patterning by parents is not responsible for homosexuality. In any case, nowadays, with androgynous fashions in clothes, hair and even make-up, outward appearance is less significant. Even in later life, cross-dressing (transvestitism) has nothing to do with homosexuality.

All we really know about the cause of homosexuality is that we know nothing at all. We are absolutely ignorant about why the common sexual attraction for the opposite sex often appears to be absent or less strong in gays and lesbians. It is just possible that the level of hormones in the mother's blood at some stage during her pregnancy affects the sexual orientation of her child when he or she reaches puberty, but even that has to be proved. However, we do now at least know enough to realize that it is not an 'illness', and not something that can or needs to be 'cured'.

Is it *safe*?

A mere inclination to prefer relations with members of the same sex is certainly safe. It is what homosexuals actively *do* with one another than can be so very unsafe, particularly with regard to fellatio and anal intercourse (see page 40 and below).

ANAL INTERCOURSE

Anal intercourse, known in legal terms as 'buggering', consists of inserting the penis into the partner's anus. This of course and inevitably is one of the ways in which homosexuals have sexual contact with one another, as it also is with heterosexuals.

The law is inconsistent about this act, because it is no longer illegal if it takes place between consenting adult males in private, but it *is* illegal for a man to have intercourse with any consenting woman (including his wife) through the anus. A man may wish to do this because the anus, being surrounded by strong muscle, is tighter than the vagina, especially if the latter has become very stretched by childbearing. Furthermore, ejaculation into the rectum, just above the anus, cannot be followed by pregnancy. But most women do not enjoy anal intercourse, even if they can have an orgasm with it.

Is it *safe*?

Strictly no. It is definitely unsafe. And it is unhealthy for the reason that germs that are harmless when confined to the anal region and to the rectum can be very harmful indeed to the penis, and can give rise to Non-specific Urethritis (NSU; see page 80) if they get into the man's urethra. If the man's urethra is already infected by any other STD, and in particular if his semen is infected with the AIDS virus HIV (see page 72), he can pass infection to his sexual partner through the rectum, whether the partner be a man or a woman. Apart from drug addicts sharing infected needles, this seems to be the way AIDS is most commonly spread, because the anus, not being as elastic as the vagina, often splits slightly, leaving a wound with open blood vessels, into which viruses and germs penetrate.

Anal intercourse should never even be contemplated without the use of a condom.

Another particular danger is the practice of a man starting intercourse by putting his penis into the woman's rectum and then coming out and inserting the penis into the vagina. He then not only risks infection of the vagina with any germs of his own that he may have in his semen or urethra, but he also takes germs that are harmless in the female rectum into the vagina, where they can be very harmful indeed. This is in fact a very risky procedure for the woman, whether a condom is used or not, and she may, as may the man himself later, develop a bladder infection called cystitis (see pages 81–82).

BISEXUALITY

The term bisexual means a person who is sometimes homosexual and sometimes heterosexual – sometimes both on the same day. Both men and women can be bisexual.

Is it *safe*?

No, it can be very unsafe indeed. A man who indulges in homosexual activity without a condom (especially in anal intercourse) is at much greater risk of acquiring a sexually transmitted disease just because a greater percentage of gays have STDs than have heterosexuals. Such a man can be a menace to his woman partner if he then has vaginal intercourse – especially, again, if he does not use a condom.

There are relatively few women bisexuals. Very few women who are exclusively lesbians have STDs, and going from a lesbian relationship to a heterosexual one only constitutes a danger if the man is infected. Even then it is difficult for a woman to pass on any infection she may have acquired to her female partner because of the necessary physical restrictions in lesbian love-making. However, bisexual men can take STDs acquired from homosexuals into the much larger heterosexual community where it will spread widely and rapidly, because of the larger number of partners involved.

PROSTITUTION

Men go to prostitutes either because they cannot find or do not want any other kind of partner, or because they want to be able to have forms of sex that their regular partner will not allow. These may include wearing unusual clothes, being beaten or being bound. Many men are relieved to have no emotional involvement in this part of their sex life.

Prostitution may seem an easy way to earn money, especially if a lot of money is needed to pay for expensive habits like drink or drugs. Very few prostitutes walk the streets soliciting, because it is now illegal and they may be arrested. About a third of the prostitutes in the UK work for a madam or pimp, who takes a part of the money received. Roughly another third work by putting discreetly worded advertisements in shop windows, or by waiting in hotel lounges. Those who walk the streets soliciting earn least and are at greatest danger. Then there are escort or massage agencies who also recruit people into prostitution, as do hostess clubs. These are nightclubs where customers are persuaded to drink at excessive prices, and, after the club closes in the early hours, may then take one of the 'staff' elsewhere for sex.

Is it *safe*?

Most emphatically no. Nobody could ever dream that prostitution is a safe form of sex, either for the clients or for the prostitutes. It is the biggest reservoir for all sexually transmissible diseases and one which is continually being replenished.

Two of the most dangerous places either to be a prostitute or to go with one are Central Africa and Bangkok in Thailand, where almost every single prostitute has an HIV infection (see page 72) with the virus of AIDS disease. Probably half of these will develop the full AIDS disease, and will die.

In Hamburg, a city which probably boasts more prostitutes than any other in northern Europe, it is claimed that a fortnightly medical inspection proves prostitutes to be free of STDs, and that any who are not cleared are prevented from working until they are.

However, this claim does not bear examination, because a prostitute may be clear at the time of inspection and the blood test may be negative for all infectious diseases. But the HIV virus takes at least several weeks and probably months to show up in a blood test, so infection will not be discovered until much more time and many more clients have come and gone. And even if a prostitute is completely clear on inspection, the very next client may bring an infection, with a whole fortnight's worth of clients then at risk, to say nothing of the risk to the prostitute.

If a woman prostitute does not insist on clients wearing a sheath and if she is only using an oral contraceptive, she has an 80 percent chance of catching gonorrhoea and at least a fair chance of having her tubes so badly infected that she is unlikely ever to be able to have children. If she uses no form of contraception and neither does the client, then she runs the risk of becoming pregnant. Many male prostitutes, most of whom are young boys willing to be passive partners for anal intercourse, are already now infected with AIDS. It is essential for male prostitutes, too, to insist that clients wear a condom.

In addition to the risk of STDs, all prostitutes run the risk of serious physical damage from clients. Some clients, of course, face the unwelcome prospect of being 'rolled', that is, having their wallets, money, and credit cards stolen.

There is no safeguard on either side in prostitution except a condom to protect against infection and pregnancy, and some additional form of contraception for women prostitutes.

There is really no 'safe' prostitute from the point of view of the client, as every prostitute who allows or has in the past allowed intercourse or fellatio without insisting that clients wear sheaths may be infected and can spread infection.

INCEST

All forms of sexual contact between close members of a family, and especially full intercourse, are illegal. Incest involves sexual relationships between members of the same family. These are usually between older men and younger girls. The prevalence of this abnormal practice is not known, but it has been guessed that some form of sexual relationship, often short of full intercourse, may occur in as many as ten percent of all families. Certainly the police know of very many cases of fathers having intercourse with their daughters over a period of many years, and it is next to useless to expect such adults to care about precautions against pregnancy or disease.

One of the most distressing cases I had to deal with was a 12-year-old girl brought to the antenatal clinic by her aunt, the sister of her dead mother. The girl was completely silent. I could not get a single word out of her, but did confirm the pregnancy. When she left the clinic the police were waiting outside, having arrested her father, and it was my very painful task to go to the Crown Court when he was tried for incest, to give evidence of the girl's advanced condition. She had to be given a caesarean operation as her pelvis was too small for normal childbirth, and unfortunately the baby died: so that the girl was deprived not only of her mother, but of her father for four years in prison, and the baby.

One can only imagine the mental scarring this poor young

girl suffered. The worst part of the whole case was that she told me afterwards that *she* felt guilty, because her mother had warned her before dying that the father was weak and would perhaps want the daughter to take her place 'in every way'. Although the 12-year-old could do nothing against her father's sexual advances, she still felt guilty and I am sure will feel guilty for all her life.

This guilt is one of the greatest tragedies of incest. It is nearly always young girls or young women who are forced or taken advantage of by fathers, uncles, older brothers and even grandfathers: and if they acquiesce, as they usually do, they feel guilty usually for life because they think they have helped their older male relatives to do something they know very well society will punish.

The cruelty is increased when the girls at school hear other girls talking about their experience of sex and of the fun they are getting out of having boyfriends, and they know that it is not for them. They know that there is no longer any mystery or any love. They know that they have been abused.

CHILD ABUSE

Although most adults involved in this know very well that they are doing something wrong and completely illegal, some men and women do take a perverse sexual pleasure in having intercourse with very young girls and boys. This is called paedophilia. There are a few women, too, who like to seduce young boys but this is not nearly so common as men seducing little girls. These men say they feel they are just giving love to the children. They sometimes even feel that the love they give is much greater than that the parents can give the children. There used to be until a few years ago a British Paedophilic Society where the members met to discuss their activities with one another, and there still is a trade in pornographic pictures and video films showing paedophilic acts. It it a very distorted way of thinking – indeed, a mental disorder.

4
AVOIDING PREGNANCY

This chapter is about avoiding unwanted pregnancies. However, some of the methods described will also help to avoid infection by the transmission of germs from the man to the woman, or by the man picking up germs from the woman's vagina.

What is necessary for sex to result in pregnancy
The answer may seem very obvious – intercourse. But intercourse has to be on the right day of the month, because only once a month is an egg for fertilization released from one of the two ovaries, in a process called ovulation (see pages 62–64). The ovaries take it in turn to release an egg, and one is usually released about fourteen days before the beginning of the next period.

If intercourse has taken place within six days or so before the egg is released, it is possible for the woman to become pregnant, because the sperms can live for up to six days if the circumstances in the vagina and the womb are favourable. The egg itself, however, can only live 24 hours at the most. Therefore if intercourse takes place in the five or six days before the release of the egg, or on the day in which the egg is released, pregnancy can but does not necessarily always result. If, however, intercourse takes place more than 24 hours after the egg has been released, intercourse is unlikely to result in pregnancy.

BARRIER METHODS

It is probable that sexual practices such as oral and anal sex, as well as just rubbing the penis between the lips of the vulva without entering the vagina, came about as ways of relieving sexual tension and obtaining sexual satisfaction without risking pregnancies. Anal intercourse with a woman may also be an effective way of doing this, but it is more than useless as a method of avoiding infection. This list of birth control methods is in alphabetical order. This order does NOT relate to the efficacy of any particular method of contraception.

Condom

This is one of the oldest methods of contraception. It is also known as the French letter, the sheath, a johnny, the rubber, or, in France, as the capote anglaise; but condom is the word used in the Government's pamphlet on AIDS.

It was in the sixteenth century that an Italian, Gabriel Fallopius (who discovered the purpose of the tubes that connect the ovaries with the womb and after whom they are named) described a sheath he had invented to put over the penis. It was made of linen and treated with some form of chemicals. It was designed to cover the tip of the penis. Fallopius intended it not so much for contraception as for protection against transmission of venereal diseases. It was a very imaginative step forward, even if his sheath was a little thick and cumbersome. Later the Marquis de Sevigné made a membrane sheath from a cow's intestine, and he called this goldbeater's skin. (The name derived from the prepared outside membrane of the large intestine of the ox, used by goldbeaters to lay between leaves of the metal while they beat it into gold leaf.) De Sevigné recommended his invention as 'an armour against love, gossamer against infection'. Certainly gossamer (light as a feather) animal intestine membranes were much thinner and lighter than linen sheaths. Mr or Dr Condom is believed to have lived in the reign of Charles II, when he invented a sheath made either from pigs' bladders or sheep's intestines.

For the last hundred years sheaths have been made of rubber, and the modern latex sheath is quite strong, only very rarely splitting during use. It is therefore an extremely safe and effective protection, not only to avoid pregnancy but for either partner to avoid catching any infection. It is only effective against pregnancy if it is put on before the penis touches the vulva at the entrance of the vagina. Entering the vagina and then withdrawing to put on the condom before ejaculation is not a good enough protection, because the first drop of semen may be squeezed out of the penis without the man being aware of it. That drop may contain more sperms than the rest of the whole ejaculate. It is also important to hold the condom on during withdrawal from the vagina. Otherwise, after the penis has lost its erection it slips out not only from the vagina but from the sheath itself, which is left behind, so inevitably spilling some of the semen, if only on to the lips of the vulva.

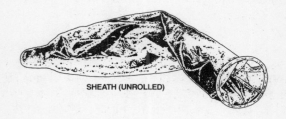

SHEATH (UNROLLED)

The sheath has to be rolled on to the erect penis before any penetration. And it has to be used every time. Too often men embark on love-making armed with just one sheath in its wrapping and do not think about the fact that they may have intercourse a second time. Some young men can have erections and can penetrate several times during a love-making session, so if intercourse is contemplated at all it is well worth while carrying three or more sheaths. Even if sex is not really contemplated, the urge may come on unexpectedly: after every year's Christmas parties, for instance, lots of girls become pregnant unintentionally and lots of men pick up infections which they then take home to their wives.

The use of condoms does not do away with the pleasure of intercourse: the security they give against risk of pregnancy and the knowledge that the semen has been trapped in the sheath may, by removing anxiety, even increase it for some. Many, but not all, do notice a lessening of sensation. This too can be a bonus for some, if it enables the man to delay his ejaculation and prolong love-making.

Diaphragm or Dutch cap

This is a dome-shaped, thin, rubber, stretchable barrier on a springy ring about $2\frac{1}{2}$–3" (55–80mm) across. The woman puts this into her vagina half an hour or so before intercourse and the rubber barrier blocks off the cervix, the neck of the womb, from the vagina. The man can have intercourse without a condom and ejaculate into the vagina, but his sperms will not go straight into her cervix as they do with normal intercourse.

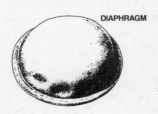

DIAPHRAGM

The rubber of the diaphragm alone does kill sperms, but it is not really sufficiently effective in doing this, so a contraceptive cream or jelly should be put around the rim as well as into the centre of the diaphragm before it is inserted. The contraceptive cream, jellies or foams not only kill sperms but also many though not all of the germs of STDs, including the virus HIV, the AIDS virus.

The diaphragm should not be removed for about six to eight hours after intercourse because it can take as long as that for the spermicidal cream to kill off all the sperms that are lying around. Once it is in position, neither of the couple will feel anything. Some girls are surprised that something as comparatively big as the diaphragm is completely unnoticeable once it has been inserted, but it really is so often forgettable that a few patients every year turn up in every gynaecological clinic, wondering why they have a discharge, only to be told that they have left a diaphragm in the vagina.

The diaphragm *should be removed* about eight hours after the last intercourse. If the couple are going to have intercourse more than once, then its protection should be added to by the further use of a contraceptive foam which is easily introduced into the vagina without disturbing the diaphragm.

There are some women who find the whole process a little bit

these pills contains 50 micrograms of oestrogen. Each variety contains a differing but fixed quantity of progestogen, the weakest being Microgynon 30, which has 30 micrograms of oestrogen and 0.15 milligrams of progestogen. The manufacturers make so many varieties because some combinations suit some women better than others.

There are pills, however, that contain only the progestogen. These sometimes go under the name of 'mini-pill'. It is a silly and misleading name because there are patients who believe, not without reason, that the word 'mini' could equally well apply to those pills with a minimum dose of the combined oestrogen and progestogen. These progestogen-only pills are taken every single day, without any breaks; and the woman does eventually acquire a fairly normal menstrual cycle of bleeding approximately once a month.

The reason why progestogen-only pills are prescribed is that there are many women who cannot take oestrogen. Some doctors believe that women with a medical history of breast cancer are more liable to develop a cancer if they are given a pill with oestrogen in it. There are other doctors who believe that the oestrogen portion of the combined pill may give rise to deep-vein thrombosis, and that women with a medical history of high blood pressure should not have the combined pill prescribed.

Many gynaecologists prefer to give what are called biphasic or triphasic pills. Biphasic pills contain two different combinations of oestrogen and progestogen in the month, and triphasic pills have three different combinations. For instance, Logynon, which is a triphasic pill, contains a slightly higher quantity of oestrogen and progestogen in the second, five-day, set of pills, which start on the seventh day of taking the pill, than in the first and third sets. The pack is made up with the days marked, so that there is no calculation needed to decide which strength pill to take on which day (see opposite). This kind of variation in the doses of hormones in the pills mimics a little better the variations that occur throughout the menstrual cycle in every woman who is not on the pill.

My own preference is to give triphasic pills such as Logynon or Trinordiol to young girls at the beginning of their sexually

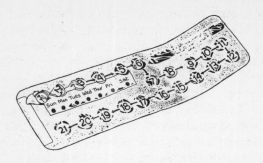

active life, because by and large they tolerate best those pills that do mimic their own natural hormone production.

The main disadvantage of the combined pill is that occasionally, with the low-dose ones, there may be some unexpected bleeding in the middle of the cycle, due to the lining of the womb building up; this bleeding is called 'break-through' bleeding. Break-through bleeding is much more common, however, with the progestogen-only pill. Even more disconcerting is a failure to have a period at all, so-called amenorrhoea.

The combined pill does not have to be taken at exactly the same time each day but the progestogen-only pill does, so it is best to keep the pack handy for some part of a daily routine. The pills are usually packaged with the day of the week written on the pack, so the girl can know whether she has taken it on, say, a Wednesday or has forgotten it. If a pill is forgotten then it is probably best to take two pills the following day, or as soon as it has been remembered.

The pill is an immensely effective method of contraception and also, surprisingly, helps to lessen the risk of inflammation in the female organs of the pelvis – the tubes and the uterus and even the ovaries – perhaps because with the pill the plug of mucus in the cervix becomes less permeable by bacteria. The pill also to a certain extent protects against cancer of the ovaries and the lining of the womb. It is just possible, however, that there is a slightly increased risk of cervical cancer and cancer of the breasts if a woman starts using the pill at a very young age and continues for very many years, but that is not proved.

One complaint that some girls on the pill have is that their breasts tend to get rather full and tender, especially in the last days of the cycle before bleeding; but this also happens in women not on the pill, and it is not a reason for stopping the pill. Other patients, especially if they are on high doses of oestrogen in the combined pill, find that their breasts do enlarge. This is fine for some girls but for others it can be a little disconcerting to have to wear a bra cup size larger than they did before taking the pill. This is a relatively minor disadvantage and the woman may cease to perceive it as one, since her partner will usually rejoice! It is rare for the breasts to become too painful to be touched, particularly on the lower-dose combined pills.

The oral contraceptive, particularly the combined oral contraceptive, is a very safe protection indeed against pregnancy, the failure rate being less than 1 in 200 women over a year (0.5 percent). It is independent of intercourse and can be taken throughout the year and it does allow women who previously had irregular periods to have absolutely regular cycles. There are great advantages therefore in the combined oral contraceptive pill.

However, there are a few reasons for not using the pill, the first being of course if the woman is already pregnant. The second is if menstration has occurred very irregularly before starting the pill, unless the doctor specifically recommends it for regulating the periods. The third is if the woman is a migraine sufferer. In a few patients a history of thrombosis may be a contra-indication to the pill, but this last contra-indication is very unlikely to be present in any young woman.

Depo-provera

This is a progestogen-only contraceptive that is given to women who are suited to it and want hormone contraception, but who can never remember to take the pill or who do not wish to be bothered with it. The progestogen is given by injection into the buttock and lasts for up to three months at a time. There are side effects, however. Menstruation may occur unexpectedly at different times. And even after the effects of the injection have worn off, it may be a long time, even up to a

year, before the girl who wants to become pregnant can
achieve it. So very careful consideration has to be given before
this form of hormone contraception is used.

For women who have had two or three children, however,
and definitely want a gap of a year or two before conceiving
again, it can be a very useful contraceptive. It has none of the
risks of the IUD, of making infection more likely, and none of
the bother of having to remember to take the pill every day. But
it is not prescribed very frequently, because some girls and
women who have it get depressed and others get annoyed with
the fact that they really do not know when they are going to
have a period. One patient said she had 'menstrual chaos' and
would not agree to having another injection. On the other
hand, some women would have no other contraceptive than
this, because of the advantages of not having to do anything
themselves and because their periods were much lighter, even
if they did come irregularly.

Douching

This is an old-fashioned and awkward contraceptive method. It
consists of running into the vagina a solution of water mixed
with an antiseptic like permanganate of potash or vinegar. It is
necessary to have a rubber or plastic bag containing the
antiseptic attached to a tube with a nozzle on one end that will
go into the vagina; the other end of the bag is attached to a
water tap. The woman sits or squats in a bath, on a bidet or even
on the lavatory seat and the bag must be held higher than the
vagina. Once the nozzle is inserted into the vagina, the tap is
turned on and the solution should reach high enough into the
vagina to wash it clean of its contents. If the tube and tap seem
too much of a complication, it is possible to fill a very large
rubber bulb, shaped like a pear, with the antiseptic solution, to
insert its nozzle into the vagina and, squeezing the bulb, to
wash out the semen that way.

As a contraceptive method it is pretty useless. Some semen
may be left in the vagina and anyway some sperms may already
have been ejaculated right into the opening of the cervix and
have gone up out of reach of the solution. Your grandmother
may have douched, but then she did not mind if she had seven

children, she only wanted a little less chance of having an eighth. But today nobody who seriously wants to practise birth control would use a douche. Furthermore, if there are air bubbles in the solution there is an increased risk of any infection present being pushed up from the vagina into the womb, especially using the rubber bulb.

Some doctors do prescribe douching as a treatment for some vaginal infections, and there are a few others who recommend it in cases of infertility where the woman wants to become pregnant: douching with a solution of bicarbonate of soda before intercourse cleans the vagina, makes it healthier for the sperms and may give them a better chance of fertilizing an egg.

Intra-uterine devices (IUDs)

These used to be called 'the coil', or, to borrow the term the French used, the sterilette, a coiled-up little roll of plastic put into the womb to inhibit pregnancy.

It is not a very good method of contraception for women who have never had a baby or have never been pregnant. There are two reasons for this. Firstly, because as the cervix is narrower before pregnancy or childbirth, there is more difficulty in inserting the IUD and a greater risk of perforating the uterus. Secondly, as IUDs are associated with an increased incidence of infection in the uterus and the Fallopian tubes, there is an increased risk of sterility, which is harder on someone who has never been pregnant (unless they never, ever, want to have a child) than on someone who has already got a family.

However, even girls who have never been pregnant do have them fitted if they really cannot face taking hormones at all. For instance, one of the leading ballet dancers in one of the London companies refused to take the pill because she said that every kind of pill she had tried made her breasts feel heavier. She persuaded her gynaecologist to fit her with an intra-uterine device. Her womb was small and therefore a small device had to be chosen, shaped like the number 7 and consisting of a plastic core with some copper wound round the stem. But it was put in and she quite happily continued dancing.

Progestasert device

There is a newer, T-shaped intra-uterine device that instead of having copper wound round the core has a little plastic tube as the upright stem of the T. This tube contains a small quantity of progestogen which is released very slowly day-to-day through its walls. The progestogen goes on being released for about a year to eighteen months. The quantity is so small that there are no general hormone effects on the body.

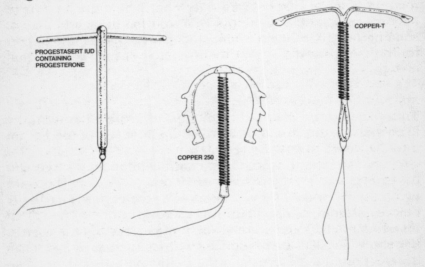

PROGESTASERT IUD CONTAINING PROGESTERONE

COPPER 250

COPPER-T

Effectiveness Nobody is quite sure yet how intra-uterine contraceptive devices work. They probably do allow the spermatozoa to go up into the uterus and meet the egg in the tube, but then they probably prevent the fertilized egg from getting a foothold in the wall of the uterus and implanting there and growing. The fertilized egg just dies off and comes out with the next period. The risks of pregnancy with the device inserted correctly, checked a month or so after insertion, and again regularly every year, are very small indeed. About two out of every 100 women who wear the device for a year and have very regular intercourse may become pregnant. Added together that means 100 years of regular intercourse can produce one or at the most two chances of pregnancy, a risk countless couples feel is not too great to take. It means that of 1000 women who are fitted with the device and have intercourse regularly, perhaps ten or fifteen, or even in a very bad year 20, may become pregnant.

Disadvantages   Intra-uterine devices are accepted and in fact enjoyed by at least three-quarters of the women to whom they have been fitted, because they do not in any way interfere with sexual pleasure and women are quite unaware that they are wearing them. They may, however, experience heavier periods. Just occasionally, too, the man can during intercourse feel the end of the thread which is fixed as a tail to the device (to facilitate its removal when its time comes for renewal or if pregnancy is desired). If this happens the doctor who has inserted the device can always cut the tail shorter.

The biggest disadvantage of the device, as compared with the pill, is that while the contraceptive pill tends to make it less likely for an infection to go up from the vagina into the womb, the IUD makes it more likely. The tail of the device acts as a kind of wick, encouraging any infection that may be present in the vagina to go up into the womb. Because of this and because of the many legal actions against one firm making intra-uterine devices, wrongly claiming the IUD as a cause of infection rather than a channel for it, this firm has stopped manufacturing and marketing the Copper Seven. The Copper T, however, is still on the market.

Morning-after pill

If a woman has had unprotected intercourse and the man has ejaculated inside her, or he even thinks he has, she is at risk of having a possibly unwanted pregnancy. Fortunately there are two fairly effective ways of making sure that a pregnancy does not develop, provided that a doctor is consulted within 72 hours of the unprotected intercourse.

The first method is known as the 'morning-after' pill. It is specially designed and contains the same hormones as the ordinary contraceptive pill but in larger doses. Two pills are taken immediately they have been obtained from a chemist on a prescription from a doctor (they can only be obtained by prescription) and another two pills are taken twelve hours later.

The 'morning-after' pill is marketed under the initials PC4. The initials stand for post-coital and the number 4 stands for the four pills in the pack.

The only trouble with these rather strong pills is that they do sometimes make women feel rather nauseated and they may even be sick. They are, however, about 90-95 percent successful in preventing pregnancy. The sooner they are taken after intercourse the more likely they are to be successful.

Another method of avoiding pregnancy even after unprotected intercourse is for a doctor to insert into the womb an intra-uterine device (IUDs; see pages 59–61) to cause temporary sterility. The IUD can be effective even if it is inserted as much as four, or perhaps even five, days after unprotected intercourse. So in some cases the stable door can be locked even though it might seem that the horse has been given every opportunity to bolt!

Safe period or rhythm method

When some religions raised strong objections to barrier and other methods of contraception, the 'safe period' was allowed instead. This means that sexual intercourse takes place on days where it is thought the woman cannot become pregnant. Until recently the method was reliable only for women who were very regular in their periods, and it is still in fact so unreliable for some women that doctors call it the 'Russian roulette' method. But now that women know how to chart and understand their temperature every morning they can have a fairly good idea of when they have ovulated.

The temperature, taken in the early morning before putting anything else in the mouth, is lower in the first half of the menstrual cycle before ovulation takes place than in the second half of the cycle after ovulation. This is due to the presence in the bloodstream of a hormone, progesterone, which is secreted by the ovary only after ovulation and until menstruation starts. The menstrual cycle is the interval of days between the first day of the period and the first day of the next period. Because sperm can live for five or six days and the egg for only one day, if intercourse takes place five or six days before ovulation the woman can still become pregnant.

Therefore, once ovulation has happened, intercourse is safe enough 24 hours later.

Another way a woman can tell when she has ovulated is that at the time of ovulation she produces much mucus and can feel the mucus coming down the vagina to her vulva. Not very many women do notice this unless their attention has been drawn to it, but then quite a lot do become conscious of this extra, clear, fluid mucus appearing in the vulva exactly half way between the first day of one period and the first day of the next. It is very unlikely for a woman to become pregnant if intercourse takes place later than two to three days after this extra fluid has been passed, because there will be no egg present to be fertilized. Anyhow, later in the month the mucus in the neck of the womb (the cervix) becomes too thick to allow sperms through.

Since some women cannot be certain about exactly which day they will ovulate, the rhythm method may fail them. The effectiveness of the rhythm method at present varies between 20 percent failure and 2 percent failure. A 20 percent failure means that 20 out of every 100 using the method for a year will become pregnant. The rhythm method is more reliable after ovulation has finished, which is after the extra amount of mucus has come through the vulva. It can also be relied on in the first eight or nine days of the cycle if another method, such as a barrier like the condom or the diaphragm, is used later on in the first half of the cycle. It is no bad thing to use two methods, provided the diaphragm is used in the first half of the cycle together with a contraceptive cream, jelly or foam. This substance could be used by itself in the second half of the cycle, if reliance is going to be placed on the rhythm method; and the likelihood of pregnancy is still further reduced without the nuisance of having to insert the diaphragm.

There is now a new dip-stick method for testing a woman's first morning specimen of urine which shows whether a certain hormone has been released. If it has, it is strongly probable that she will ovulate within the next 36 hours or so. The test looks for the luteinizing hormone which the body starts producing about 36 hours before ovulation. The test was designed to enable women who were trying to have babies to know when to have intercourse, but it can be used almost as effectively as a method of telling women when to avoid intercourse. It is a rather expensive way of testing for the safe days of the month.

Spermicides
These can be creams, tablets, vaginal suppositories or jellies. They have the great advantage that they are easy to obtain and do not require a doctor to advise at all on how to use them. Their great disadvantage, however, is that used alone they are utterly unreliable and only slightly reduce the chance of pregnancy, say by about 50 percent, which is certainly not good enough for those who want to have intercourse but emphatically do not want a pregnancy. Yet they are invaluable, both as contraception and for killing germs of STDs, if they are used together with a condom or a diaphragm, or used together with an oral contraceptive pill.

HYSTERECTOMY

Hysterectomy consists of removal of the womb. A woman without a womb cannot, of course, become pregnant. But hysterectomy should never be used as a form of contraception even when all other methods have failed. It is a very major operation and should be performed only when there are other good medical reasons for it, such as fibroids. Not all women who have a hysterectomy realize that they are sterile for ever, but they are.

STERILIZATION

This is carried out in women by cutting the Fallopian tubes, or in men by cutting the vasa, the tubes from the testis at the top of the scrotum. It is not a method recommended for young couples, because although there have been successful reversals of sterilization, the operation is a big one. The only people who really should be sterilized are those who are absolutely certain that they never, ever, ever want a child or another child, and are old enough not to be likely to change their minds.

TERMINATION

Provided a pregnancy is really unwanted, termination can be obtained relatively easily now in many centres in the UK. There are advertisements posted in many areas giving the telephone numbers of charity organizations that arrange for terminations of pregnancy. The best system, however, is to go to your own doctor and ask for advice. Not every unintentional pregnancy needs to be terminated. For instance, even if it is unexpected and unplanned, a pregnancy in a good stable relationship should continue, provided that all the other circumstances are reasonable. The fact that the pregnancy is not planned is no reason at all for terminating it.

Good reasons for terminating pregnancy are: bad health; the possibility of having a disease that can be passed on; mental breakdown or even great stress; being deserted by the boyfriend or perhaps not even knowing which one it is; and being under the threat of being turned out of the home by an irate parent.

The decision to have a termination is a very serious one and should be talked over if possible with the family doctor or with a counsellor in one of the clinics. Two doctors have to sign the form recommending termination. This is the green Certificate A. At least one of the doctors should have examined the girl carefully to make sure firstly that she is pregnant, secondly how far on she is pregnant, and thirdly that there is no infection in her vagina that could be pushed up into her uterus and tubes. Once the form is signed, arrangements are made for her to attend a hospital or clinic for the termination.

Most National Health Service hospitals should provide a rapid termination of pregnancy service which should be available free, quickly and preferably as a day procedure, provided the pregnancy has lasted less than twelve weeks. Most terminations are carried out under a general anaesthetic.

In National Health Service hospitals, as well as in charity clinics run by pregnancy advisory services, there are usually a lot of girls having terminations on the same day and the doctors doing them have become extremely skilled. If a general anaesthetic is going to be administered it is important that no food or drink should be taken in the twelve hours before the operation, or, if it is going to be in the afternoon, in the six or seven hours before the operation.

The girl undresses and, most important, empties her bladder just before the operation. She is put to sleep with an injection in her arm and the contents of her womb are sucked out with a little vacuum apparatus attached to a plastic tube that is passed into the neck of the womb. This has been stretched by the doctor to allow the correct sized plastic tube to be passed. The size of tube depends on the duration of the pregnancy.

This is an extremely effective way of terminating a pregnancy in the early stages, and the complication rate, now that the doctors have become so skilled at it, is very low indeed. Usually the girl is able to go home three or four hours after the termination, but she may have to stay in overnight, particularly if there has been a lot of bleeding, which can occasionally happen. It is important, of course, to be sure that effective contraception is used immediately afterwards. The pill can be taken from the day after the termination and intercourse can usually be resumed about ten days later.

If the above account makes termination of pregnancy seem dead easy and something not to be thought seriously about, that is a completely false impression. Many, many girls do regret having had terminations. They will put a brave front on it and pretend they are not upset, and, in fact, quite a few may not mind very much at the time. But for nearly all of them it is a loss, a matter for mourning or for regret at least. Regret may be the wrong word when termination has been very carefully considered, but mourning is certainly a correct description. Some women confess even years later how they miss the child they have allowed to be destroyed. One patient recently told me that it would have been the baby's seventh birthday approximately the day she came to see me, seven years after her pregnancy had been terminated; it was at a very early stage of the pregnancy, too. So if it is possible to see a counsellor as well as the two doctors before having a termination, that is very advisable.

Once a pregnancy has gone past the twelfth week, far greater skills are needed to terminate it, and it becomes important not only to attend a good hospital or charity clinic but to consider very carefully indeed with the doctors and social workers or counsellors there whether it is not better to allow the pregnancy to continue. Unfortunately some pregnancies have to be terminated because tests have shown that the baby is not developing normally. That is a very sad state of affairs, but termination then is much better than allowing a grossly abnormal child to be born.

TESTING FOR PREGNANCY

Even with the best will in the world some forms of contraception may fail or be forgotten, and some girls may find themselves pregnant.

How does a girl know she is pregnant? Well, she may have her suspicions even before she misses a period, because she may have gone off coffee or some other favourite food. As soon as she is late, she can go to her doctor and ask for a urine test, or she can buy in a chemist's shop one of the many tests now available to see whether she is pregnant. Discover 2 is a good one, because it gives her two chances of testing urine (passed first thing in the morning, so that it is concentrated) for the hormones that are evidence of her being pregnant.

These home kit tests are very reliable, but if the test is negative and the girl still has not had a period a week or so later, she can repeat the test. A new one on the market is called Clear Blue, and that seems to be a very safe test. The chemist may equally sell others, or he may be willing to do the test himself with the girl's first morning specimen of urine. Doctors can also take blood and have it examined for the homone even when the period is just a day or two late. Sometimes the hormone test comes up positive a day or so before the last day of the cycle, but it is more reliable when performed a week after a period has been missed.

5
SEXUALLY TRANSMITTED DISEASES (STDs)

This chapter contains a list of sexually transmissible diseases, which are those infections usually transmitted by sexual intercourse but not otherwise contagious. Fortunately, all of them are curable with the exception of herpes, which is really not a very serious illness and AIDS, which is.

Many people when reading details about a disease, whether it is sexually transmitted or any other, such as a stomach ulcer, imagine that they must have it – medical students do it all the time. Most people then find they do not have any disease at all. But there are today too many sufferers from STDs, so at the risk of scaring a few people unnecessarily the diseases will be described.

Anybody who is worried can easily check whether their worries are justified by going to a 'special' clinic. Almost all large hospitals have these clinics specially for the diagnosis and treatment of STDs. In most hospitals they are now called 'genito-urinary medicine' clinics (GUMs).

So, if a man thinks he may have caught something sexually and has, say, some trouble in passing water, or if a woman has an unusual discharge and is worried that she may have caught something, it is very wise indeed to seek professional help quickly from one of these clinics or from your own doctor. It is so much better than letting an illness incubate until it is more difficult to treat.

How does a person suspect he or she may have caught an STD? By the symptoms, things that the patient himself or herself feels, and the signs, things that the patient or doctor sees as characteristic of the disease. The commonest symptoms, apart from the nuisance of the discharge and even the need to wear extra protection, are soreness, pain or a scalding sensation on passing urine. The commonest signs are discharge, which means something coming out of the tip of the penis or down the vagina and which stains the clothing; or spots, sores and lumps (see pages 85 and 87).

A discharge may be yellow and frothy, as in the condition of trichomonas; or colourless but smelly as in the condition of gardnerella; or white and curdy as in the condition of candida; or yellow and accompanied by a burning sensation in passing urine as in gonorrhoea; or sometimes blood-stained as in carcinoma-in-situ, which means a pre-cancerous tumour which is strictly localized, that is, not spreading. The name comes from the Greek word for cancer and the Latin words for in position.

Pain may occur only on passing urine, but there is very often a continuous nagging ache made much worse on intercourse. Both men and women may suffer dyspareunia, as pain during intercourse is called. It is especially likely to be felt when infection involves the Fallopian tubes in women.

A raised temperature, raised pulse rate and a general feeling of illness may occur when the infection is most active. The symptoms and signs vary from disease to disease.

It is common for two infections to exist in one patient at the same time. For instance, a large proportion of those who have gonorrhoea also have a trichomonas infection. If only one is treated, that illness will be cured, but not the other one which may need different drugs.

Sexually transmitted diseases can be caught in a few other ways than by intercourse. For instance, both gardnerella and trichomonas can, though very rarely, be caught from swimming pools; but most pools are adequately sterilized, especially on sunny days where the sun kills germs (bacteria). Jacuzzis, however, may not be so safe. In those, the water is churned up so fast that if a man or a woman has a discharge and it leaks into the water, it may be transmitted to a girl sitting nearby in the jacuzzi, because the vagina is often open and the water bubbling away can enter the lower part of it. Men are very unlikely to catch illnesses in jacuzzis, but some of the STDs, such as perhaps gardnerella or candida, may very occasionally be caught that way. Although jacuzzis nearly always have a fair amount of chlorine mixed in with the water so that one can smell it, the chlorine may not be quite strong enough to kill all viruses and germs.

Although it really is virtually impossible to catch a sexually transmitted disease from a toilet seat, one may occasionally be caught from the lavatory pan. Many of the germs mentioned in this chapter can survive only too well in the water at the bottom of the lavatory. Patients often say that they never sit on the lavatory seat, but it is not uncommon for water that is splashed up from the lavatory pan to touch the vulva or anus and this could cause an infection. It is almost impossible for anyone to sit on a lavatory and not occasionally have this happen, even if the little drops are so small that they cannot be felt touching the body. When one doctor's wife (also his receptionist) caught trichomonas, he was furious, and accused the laboratory of mixing the specimen obtained from his wife with that from another patient. This was not so. A culture dish filled with a culture medium was placed upside down supported by two rods across the lavatory seat in his surgery, which was used by the patients as well as by his wife. To the doctor's and everybody else's surprise, many germs splashed up when the lavatory was flushed. So although STDs are usually caught by sexual activity, some people can be infected innocently.

It is sensible to flush the lavatory before sitting down in any strange place and only to sit down after the whole perturbance in the water at the bottom of the pan has settled. Of course, the lavatory should be flushed after use as well as before. Even in your own home, if strangers use the lavatory it is a good tip to flush it once or twice before using it yourself.

There is no place for amateur treatment of genital infections. It is a doctor's job and the doctors who work in the special clinics freely welcome clients (as their patients are called) and encourage anyone to come in who is worried that they have caught something. They welcome people coming in even if they have no disease, because it is nice to be able to reassure somebody who is worried that there is nothing wrong, nothing there that is going to turn into something worse or is going to be passed on to somebody else. No doctor in one of these clinics will ever tell a client that he or she is wasting time.

The special clinics work in strict confidence. Even your own

GP will not know you have been to one, unless you yourself tell him or her. There is no need to have a letter from your doctor to go to a genito-urinary clinic.

Many of the people who turn up at GUM clinics are worried that they have acquired an STD previously because they have been reminded of a long-past affair by seeing something in a book, in a film, or on television. Then the worry nags at them. They should go to a doctor or to a clinic and find out if they have any good cause for worrying.

Other patients are worried that they may recently have caught something, even though they may not have had any sexual contact with an infected person – they just want to be sure. Well, you cannot catch STDs from drinking from cups that have not been properly washed, nor from shaking hands, nor from eating from plates that have been used by infected people, nor even from sharing a bed without close contact such as intercourse or French kissing, or even from wearing somebody else's clothes, except perhaps underwear that has not been washed. Even in that way no serious disease can be transmitted, although occasionally there may be a chance of picking up a fungus infection or crabs (see pages 76–77 and 86–87).

STDs are most often passed by unprotected full sexual intercourse, but other forms of sexual activity, such as oro-genital sex and especially anal sex, can result in one person infecting another with an STD unless a condom is used.

The organs most often affected are the genital organs; and the symptoms that the patients feel are quite often related to the passing of urine, hence the name 'genito-urinary medicine'. Passing urine may be painful, may be difficult, or may occur far too often.

STDs are so common that one women in 50 under the age of 24 will be affected every year, and of all age groups, one in 100 women in the UK will certainly have an STD in any one year. Heterosexual or bisexual men, who generally have more partners, are more likely to catch STDs. Homosexuals who are without a stable relationship to restrain them may have many more partners still and may therefore be more exposed to STDs.

The most common long-term effect of an STD is infertility,

due to chronic pelvic inflammatory disease, but it can be avoided by early effective treatment. Few people realize how easily and quickly sexually transmitted diseases are 100 percent cured. Only herpes and AIDS still cannot be cured, but herpes can be kept well under control.

Here is a list of some of the most common sexually transmissible diseases treated by the special clinics. This list is in alphabetical order. This order does NOT relate to the frequency with which any particular STD may occur.

AIDS
candida, or thrush
cervical cancer,
    CIN I, CIN II, CIN III
    carcinoma-in-situ
        (a pre-cancerous condition
        probably caused by a virus)
cystitis

gardnerella
genital warts
gonorrhoea
herpes genitalis
scabies and pediculosis,
    or crabs
syphilis
trichomonas

AIDS
(Acquired Immune Deficiency Syndrome)

The biggest turn-off for promiscuous sex has undoubtedly been AIDS. This illness was a mystery when it first appeared in about 1980, but later it was realized that it was caused by a virus, HIV, the Human Immunedeficiency Virus, also called the HTLV 3 virus, which stands for Human T Lymphotrophic Virus, type 3.

The T in HTLV stands for the T lymphocyte, a cell which originates in the thymus below the thyroid and during childhood helps establish immunological responses. It is these cells which are so important for the body's whole immune system and which are knocked out by AIDS. The thymus atrophies with age and is almost non-existent in adults, but immune cells are made by other parts of the body's immune system, such as B lymphocytes, which is why AIDS is not rapidly fatal.

HIV can be in the bloodstream without any signs or symptoms of AIDS. It is most often transmitted from sexual partner to sexual partner, more often from one homosexual man to another but also from bisexual men to their female partners, although it must be said that the vagina is apparently more resistant to HIV than the rectum.

AIDS is a terrible condition because, as its name suggests, it stops the sufferer from being able to resist certain other infections. One of these is a form of pneumonia, and AIDS victims tend to have pneumonia more easily than any other single illness because they have no longer got the mechanism, called the immunity, to fight the pneumonia germ. With heavy doses of antibiotics, however, they often recover from the initial attack of AIDS, but maybe have subsequent attacks over several years.

Certain forms of cancer, and particularly one vicious skin cancer known as kaposi sarcoma, which is another viral infection, also seem to develop more easily in AIDS victims than in other people, as do terrible diseases such as inflammation of the brain (encephalitis), inflammation of the eyes leading to blindness, and chronic nose infections.

Infected mothers can give AIDS to their children but otherwise it is always transmitted by a blood path. By this is meant that if a passive homosexual who allows others to have anal intercourse with him has a little cut in his anus or rectum into which the HIV-infected semen of his partner can flow, then he will be infected through the blood in the cut. It is also transmitted among drug addicts by sharing infected needles.

The incubation period after infection with HIV may be very long indeed, even up to two or three years. Because the incubation period is so very long it was thought initially that only about one in four people who had acquired HIV developed AIDS, but in fact AIDS does develop in larger percentages of people with HIV than was expected. Fortunately, not everybody with HIV infection develops full-blown AIDS.

It was the death from AIDS of the film star Rock Hudson and his public admission that he was homosexual that principally brought this awful disease to the public's notice, who quite rightly demanded more information about it and instruction in methods of avoiding it. The Government in the UK has reacted positively to this very real danger by distributing information leaflets, as have governments in some other countries. Although some of this publicity has been labelled as scaremongering, it really is not. AIDS is a frightful disease and it is essential to get the message across that the more sexual partners a person has, and the less protection in the form of condoms that person has with these multiple sexual partners, the more chance there is of catching the disease.

As yet AIDS is not widespread in the UK but if there are increasing numbers of AIDS sufferers and if people have intercourse without adequate protection, then gradually the risk of picking up the virus and later developing AIDS will increase.

Bisexual men put the wide, as opposed to the homosexual, community at most risk, particularly if they travel in countries where AIDS is more prevalent and have intercourse there without a condom with a prostitute, man or woman. If a man is infected but does not know it because the incubation period is so long, comes home, and has intercourse with his wife, he faces the risk not only of developing AIDS himself but of transmitting HIV to his wife and perhaps to his unborn children.

If the first sign is a light attack of pneumonia and the doctor attending the patient is not aware that he must test for the presence of AIDS, the diagnosis may be missed and the opportunity to treat that particular manifestation of AIDS is gone.

Quite clearly, there are three important ways in which to deal with AIDS. The first consists of several choices: to avoid acquiring AIDS either by avoiding intercourse with more than one reliable partner; or by insisting that the partner, if a man, wears a condom, and wearing a condom yourself; or by avoiding all intercourse, either vaginal or rectal or oral.

The second step is being taken by the medical profession: they are searching as hard as possible to find a vaccine against the spread of AIDS, so that anybody at risk can be vaccinated for protection, and in time the disease will be completely wiped out. This is perfectly possible, as with the vaccine that was developed against smallpox. It was finally perfected and after along time it eradicated the disease completely throughout the world.

Thirdly, the most important step is to find a cure for those people who are already infected with AIDS. Not only governments but the pharmaceutical profession as well as doctors are searching for ways of treating the established disease.

There is little doubt that the journalists exaggerated the seriousness of herpes in the late 1970s. Herpes is not in any way a killer disease, but AIDS is once it has been acquired, and that is something very serious indeed. The number of AIDS victims *is* multiplying very rapidly and therefore the publicity about it is justified, in order to try to avoid its spread throughout the population. But people are perhaps more frightened than they need be.

AIDS *cannot* be passed from one child to another in class. AIDS *cannot* be caught from drinking from cups that have been used by infected victims. AIDS *cannot* be caught from mosquito bites or any other insect bites. AIDS *cannot* be caught by kissing unless there is an open sore on or inside the mouth with a little blood on it. AIDS *can*, however, be caught by unprotected sexual intercourse, particularly by anal intercourse or fellatio. AIDS *can* be transmitted from a mother to a child. AIDS *can* be caught by using infected needles for drugs.

AIDS could at one time be passed by being accidentally injected into the bloodstream of people like haemophiliacs, who need blood products to help their blood to clot, and people who are having blood transfusions.

Extremely secure screening has now eradicated the risk of medical transfusion of infected blood, but many patients have become so worried about this risk that they are increasingly avoiding blood transfusions even when these are really necessary during operations. They should no longer harbour this fear. Apart from blood screening, many categories of potential blood donors are excluded from giving blood at all. They include all active homosexuals; all patients whose blood shows evidence of HIV; the sexual partners of people known to have HIV or who have had intercourse in red light districts where HIV is prevalent; and drug addicts, particularly those who use drugs intravenously. Needles can only be sterilized to kill the HIV with great difficulty and unfortunately drug addicts, in particular heroin addicts, do tend to share needles or to use unsterilized needles.

CANDIDA ALBICANS, ALSO CALLED MONILIA OR THRUSH

It is possible for this fungus infection to reside more or less permanently in a woman's vagina doing no harm. It may be virtually without symptoms, as it is usually a very mild infection, but it can flare up.

The healthy vagina contains a lot of 'good' germs. The most common health-giving germ in the vagina is called Doederlein's bacillus; it keeps the vagina mildly acid and so keeps all the other germs under proper control. For instance, the lowest part of the vagina almost certainly has in it some of the coliform germs that inhabit the back passage, something which is particularly likely if the woman's personal hygiene is not perfect. The coliform germs and the candida fungus are kept in check when there are enough Doederlein's bacilli present.

If for any reason the Doederlein's bacilli are reduced in number, or killed off completely, as happens when antibiotics are given for an infection such as bronchitis, other infections like candida may not be hit by the antibiotics and so have a chance to multiply and cause symptoms. The vagina and vulva then become red and inflamed, hot, itchy and irritating. The vulva may become too sore to sit on. Intercourse, needless to say, becomes very painful indeed. The partner will not necessarily have or catch the candida, especially if he is circumcized, although if he is uncircumcized some dormant candida may be found under his foreskin.

Candida is especially likely to occur in women who have diabetes. It simply loves the sugar that is passed in the urine and flourishes in the moisture around the opening to the urethra, spreading backwards along the vulva and upwards into the vagina.

Candida can occur in very young children, who may acquire

it from their mothers during delivery or from anyone handling a baby with it who has not washed her hands adequately before handling another baby. Babies have candida in the mouth and in the skinfolds more often than in the genital organs.

Doctors diagnose candida under the microscope, although most experienced doctors can recognize it from the appearance of the white curd-like discharge. The treatment for it is with pessaries and creams, the most effective being Canesten, Gynodaktarin, and Ecostatin. There is also a tablet that can be taken to keep candida under control if it affects other organs than the vagina, vulva or penis.

Warning The treatment for candida by antifungal creams and jellies cannot be used at the same time as diaphragms or sheaths, as the base in which the medical substances are dissolved destroys rubber. The contraceptive effect of the diaphragm or the sheath is lost and pregnancy may result if reliance is placed on any barrier method involving rubber while undergoing treatment for candida.

CERVICAL CANCER AND THE PRE-CANCEROUS CONDITIONS OF CIN I, CIN II, CIN III, AND CARCINOMA-IN-SITU

Towards the end of 1986, a BBC *Panorama* programme talked about cancer of the cervix. A Dr Albert Singer pointed out that in most cases cervical cancer could be considered a sexually transmitted illness. Singer, with teams of doctors and scientists at the Royal Northern, the Whittington and Guy's hospitals in London, made the discovery that many, but not all, very early cervical cancers were associated with a virus infection. One virus that might increase the risk of cancer is the herpes virus, although it is not certain that it will always do this. Another is the genital wart virus or HPV (see page 83). It is associated with the presence of warts on the penis, on the vulva or in the lower part of the vagina. A man can transmit HPV in his semen without himself suffering anything at all. Only one of the many viruses that are found in warts, in the vulva or in smears taken from the cervix will give rise to cancer. It is called HPV 16.

Cancer is a very serious disease when it is fully established in the cervix. It is, however, completely curable in the early stages, which should be easy to diagnose. At first there are just slight changes in the cells on the surface of the cervix. Later there are more pronounced changes, and later still there are other alterations that do predict to the trained eye that a full cancer could develop.

The first thing that must be emphasized is that the earliest changes, which are known as CIN I and II, may reverse themselves without any treatment. The letters CIN stand for the rather technical words Cervical Intraepithelial Neoplasia, meaning changes in the cells on the surface or just under the surface of the cervix.

Cancer of the cervix, while it certainly is a killer disease, is not that common. What is disturbing is that although fewer older women are now dying of it, more young ones are, and these have usually got cervical cancer as a result of being infected with the virus.

The age at which women are likely to show evidence of cervical cancer is 35 and over, but increasingly and probably because of promiscuity, younger women are developing the earlier stages. Fortunately the smear test, also known as the Papanicoloau test, can pick up these very early stages of the conditions which could develop into cervical cancer, and which are therefore called pre-cancerous.

The Government has now become aware that it was shortsighted to organize smear tests only for the over 35s and only every five years, when so many younger women were developing early cancers in the easily treatable stages. Any woman who has been having intercourse for three years should certainly have an annual smear test and perhaps also the newer colposcopy test. In some countries such tests are automatic if a woman goes to a gynaecologist.

The colposcope is simply a pair of binoculars that magnify the view from about a foot away from the cervix. The colposcope test really involves little more that an ordinary vaginal examination. That means the passage of a speculum, a metal instrument all gynaecologists routinely use, particularly when inserting intra-uterine contraceptive devices or taking smears for detection of early cancer, or taking swabs from the cervix to detect whether any infection is sexually transmitted or not. The colposcope itself is not put into the vagina but is adjusted so that the doctor, sitting in front of the vulva, can view the neck of the womb. He washes the cervix with a certain solution to make it show up still better and can see very clearly what it looks like under magnification. He may even be able to take tiny pieces absolutely painlessly from the cervix to send to the laboratory for more thorough investigation under a greater magnification and this will pick up any very early cancers very effectively. Colposcopies should be repeated whenever the smear test shows anything suspicious at all; some doctors believe they should be repeated every three to five years.

These early stages of pre-cancerous conditions of the cervix are easily treated: by freezing them away absolutely painlessly by a technique known as cryosurgery, or burning them away by a hot wire or small metal ball, known as a cautery, usually done under general anaesthetic. Lasers are also used now, either under a general anaesthetic or without anaesthetic at all. Lasers vaporize but do not burn the tissues. The doctor who has been specially trained to use a colposcope can not only see which cells have to be destroyed but can train the laser beam very accurately on to the diseased tissues. Healthy tissue grows in place of the cells that have either been frozen, burned, or vaporized with laser. This has been a dramatic improvement in the very early treatment of the preliminary stages of cervical cancer, and has already saved thousands of women's lives throughout the world.

If the early stages of cervical cancer have been neglected, more serious methods of treatment have to be undertaken to get rid of the disease. The first of these is treatment with radioactive substances like radium, although radium itself is not often now used. Radioactive caesium is more commonly employed and the treatment is given by specially trained doctors called radiotherapists. The radioactive substance is always inserted under a general anaesthetic. Operations for the removal of the womb (hysterectomy) are also undertaken and are very effective indeed when the cancer is an early one.

Cures of at least 80 percent are being obtained in the early stages of invasive cancer. In the pre-cancerous stages, however, the cure rate is nearer 100 percent, even without the use of radioactive substances or major surgery. Lasers are very effective and although some patients do relapse they can be treated again and if necessary a third time with further laser applications or with freezing or burning.

Cancer of the womb is not always a sexually transmitted condition. Publicity that says it is is exaggerated. It was certainly a good idea to try to tell the public that promiscuity was the reason for much cancer, but if a woman develops a cancer or pre-cancerous condition of the cervix she should not automatically accuse her partner of having been unfaithful to her, or blame herself for previous indiscretions. What is not exaggerated, however, is that smoking makes it more likely for a women to develop cervical cancer, because somehow her immunity to cancer *is* reduced by cigarette smoking.

CHLAMYDIA TRACHOMATIS, OR NSU

This will occasionally cause a discharge in women and commonly an urethritis (infection in the water passage) in men. It arises after unprotected intercourse with an infected partner but it can be difficult to be certain which germ is causing the inflammation, which is why it is often called non-specific urethritis (NSU), meaning no special germ. A man has pain and, sometimes, difficulty in passing urine and he needs to empty his bladder more often. There *can* be a discharge from the penis.

We do not know what makes the infection flare up. Like gardnerella in the vagina, chlamydia may stay dormant in the cervix (the neck of the womb). Very often when a patient has been treated successfully for gonorrhoea and yet some urethritis remains, it is due to undiagnosed chlamydia, and even newborn infants may occasionally be infected by it. The treatment is with antibiotics like tetracyclines.

CYSTITIS

Cystitis, an infection of the bladder, occurs very often in women who indulge in a hectic sex life particularly after an interval of some weeks or months. The germs or bacteria infecting the bladder are not necessarily transmitted from the man to the woman. A woman can become infected with her own germs because the vagina is very close to the rectum which is full of germs, particularly those that go by the name of coliforms.

If hygiene is not very good, for instance if a woman tends to wipe herself after passing a motion from the back towards the front, instead of from the front towards the back, inevitably some of the bacteria from the rectum will hang around the back part of the vulva near the urethra. Coliforms are healthy in the rectum; they are needed there. They are not healthy in the urethra and they are usually washed away when the woman passes urine.

However, coliforms may be introduced into the urethra if intercourse is clumsy, and particularly if there is some bruising of the bladder. This is especially likely to occur if the man enters the vagina from the rear. Many couples occasionaly do practise rear entry into the vagina. It does not often result in cystitis, because usually the penis goes straight up the vagina. It is only when the penis tends to be directed toward the very front of the vagina, sometimes because the woman has not flexed her hips enough, that the bladder, which is in front of the vagina, becomes bruised (see overleaf). Bruising involves breaking some of the little blood vessels in the bladder and the release of a small quantity of blood; and blood is a perfect substance to grow germs in. Hence the development of cystitis.

Every doctor knows the term 'honeymoon cystitis' because on honeymoon sexual activity is usually much more frequent than usual. Of course we all know that many couples now have sex with one another long before the honeymoon. But holidays together do give an opportunity for much more frequent and relaxed intercourse and one of the ways to prevent spoiling a

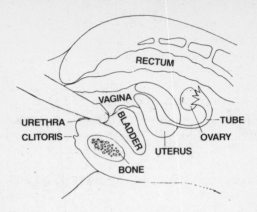

holiday, particularly if there have been previous attacks, is for the woman to ask her doctor for a mild antibiotic to take on holiday, and to swallow one or two of these tablets after sex. A good one that is better tolerated than some of the other antibiotics is Monotrim (trimethoprim). Another that contains trimethoprim together with a sulphonamide is called Septrin. This may not be quite so well tolerated but it does also act as a prevention against some other STDs.

All antibiotics require a doctor's prescription; chemists in the UK are not allowed to give out antibiotics over the counter without one. Specialists do recommend women who have had previous attacks of cystitis to drink a lot of fluids, in particular water, and also to pass urine as soon as possible after intercourse.

GARDNERELLA

This infection, which was hardly heard of before 1980, is now one of the more common STDs. It can be caught without intercourse. Many people apparently harbour the germ without having any symptoms, but occasionally something happens to make the infection active, so that a very unpleasantly smelling, often fairly colourless discharge starts. It is much more common in women than in men because the passage of urine does not flush the discharge away from the vagina as it does from the male urethra.

The gardnerella germ can be seen on cultures under a microscope. Treatment with metronidazole (Flagyl) is extremely effective. The diagnosis of gardnerella, as of all other sexually transmitted diseases, and the way each particular infection in each particular patient should be treated, *must* be decided by a doctor.

GENITAL WARTS

These are becoming commoner, both in men and women. Men with warts on their penis can give their partners warts on the vulva or in the vagina.

Warts are caused by the wart virus or the human papilloma virus (HPV). Small warts cause very little upset, but some people worry because obviously they are not normal things to have and because warts can become very large, covering almost the whole penis or the whole vulva. In this case they may make intercourse almost impossible. Certainly their presence, in whatever size, on either the penis or the vulva, is a warning that unprotected intercourse will very likely result in transmission of the infection to one's partner or partners.

It is believed that the wart virus may also be a cause of cancer of the cervix, or at least of CIN I, II or III (see pages 77–80). It is therefore very important that warts should be treated even if they are very small, and also that once they have been diagnosed regular check-ups should be carried out to be certain that there is no permanent infection and no early cancer developing. As with any other STD, the risk of spreading infection is very high if a condom is not used during sex. Unfortunately, both men and women do suffer from warts around the anus, so that a homosexual man with warts on or near his anus can certainly transmit it to any or all of his partners, as can a heterosexual woman.

The treatment of warts can take a long time. In the first place, provided the woman is not pregnant, when the treatment would be dangerous, Podophyllin is used. This is a plant extract which is painted on to the warts two or three times a week by a nurse. It has to be washed off after a few hours because otherwise it may burn the surrounding healthy skin. If Podophyllin does not work, the warts may be frozen off, or alternatively burnt off under a general anaesthetic. It is important to keep the warts completely under control and to be alert for cancer symptoms in patients who have had them.

GONORRHOEA

This is a common disease caused by a small round microbe. Initially it is always localized to the genital organs, although after a time it can cause a rise in temperature and even inflammation in the joints. The treatment for gonorrhoea has for a long time been penicillin, but now, unfortunately, there have arisen some strains of the gonorrhoea germ that have become resistant to penicillin. However, other treatments have been found and are available. Always in the end the disease is still completely curable.

In women who have caught gonorrhoea from unprotected intercourse, the vulva can become inflamed and a discharge pours out of the vagina. Underneath the back end of the vulva on each side are two glands called Bartholin's glands, and these, too, can become infected. But quite often it is the cervix, the neck of the womb, which is first infected, with pus coming from it. If the illness is not treated at this stage the infection may go up the womb and into the tubes. If if is not treated vigorously and thoroughly, blockage of the tubes may occur, leading to infertility later. If the infection of the tubes is very serious it will become an abscess, causing a high temperature and a lot of pain in the lower abdomen; if intercourse is attempted, it is excruciatingly painful. Just occasionally intercourse may cause peritonitis to develop and in some cases an infection around the liver, so-called peri-hepatitis, both making the patient very ill indeed.

Quite often, however, the woman can be infected with gonorrhoea and transmit it to her sexual partner without having any symptoms of a discharge or pain. She must, in spite of this, attend for tests once her partner realizes he is infected, because of the dangers to her. Furthermore, if she is not treated, she will continue to infect any other partners she has.

If a man has had intercourse with a woman infected with gonorrhoea without the protection of a condom he will have pus flowing from his urethra within two to six days. His penis will become inflamed. Passing water is then so painful that the French have invented the very neat term chaude-piss (hot piss) for the sensation of passing urine in the presence of a gonorrhoeal infection. So long as the man is treated at this stage he will be cured quickly. If he is not treated the initial condition may ease off, but later it will be followed by some scarring in the urethra, making it so difficult for him to pass urine that it is almost impossible. Fortunately most people are sensible enough to go for treatment quickly, so that this now rare complication does not develop.

HERPES GENITALIS

This STD has certainly caught public attention. It is not nearly as bad as many journalists make out, but it is bad enough.

There are two main herpes viruses. One causes the very common 'cold sores' that most people have at some time or other around the nose or lips during an attack of the common cold, or soon after. Another similar virus causes chickenpox, or, in many cases, shingles. The herpes virus that causes so much upset is known as Herpes Virus Hominis type II.

In a man the condition usually starts as one or two small spots on the penis, looking like blisters filled with water. These may be quite itchy. When scratched, the spot surface tears off, leaving a small ulcer, and it is in this ulcer that very many millions of the herpes virus can be found. In women the first sign is usually an itchy spot on the vulva, then another one or two more spots develop. Soon, again, these break down to form small shallow ulcers. The average ulcer is not much larger than a pinhead but if there are very many on one or other or both lips of the vulva at the same time, the condition is extremely painful, especially on passing urine.

The big trouble with herpes is not so much that it causes pain, and sometimes quite a nasty fever accompanied by a feeling of weakness, sickness and general upset as with 'flu, but because at present it is difficult to predict and prevent recurrences. This does not mean that attacks cannot be stopped. Acyclovir, a substance marketed under the name of Zovirax, is quite effective when taken by mouth or when applied as a cream to the herpes sores. The acute discomfort from herpes may last only a few days. What is known, however, is that attacks usually become less severe and more infrequent in time. Unfortunately, there is as yet no way of vaccinating to prevent its spread, as there is for diseases such as German measles.

It is because of its effects on newborn children that herpes is so feared. If an infant has become infected during its delivery through an infected cervix, vagina or vulva, it is likely to develop inflammation of the brain (encephalitis) which can leave it mentally damaged and possibly physically crippled as well.

Any woman who has been known to suffer from herpes should be examined extremely carefully during pregnancy, and especially three or four weeks before the baby is due to be born. If there is any evidence whatsoever of herpes in the vagina or the vulva it is absolutely essential for the baby to be born by caesarean operation. Such an operation, by which the baby is born through the abdomen instead of in the usual vaginal way, avoids passage through those areas where it would be likely to catch the infection.

It is the drama of the damaged child that has given the journalists such a field day and caused so much fear among people that they may catch this illness, one which initially they may not know they have. The great publicity the disease has had, and the fact that herpes can be so easily transmitted, as well as the social stigma associated with it, may have done more to persuade people that sticking to one, or at the most two or three reliable partners, is the most sensible way to live.

SCABIES AND PEDICULOSIS, OR CRABS

These are picked up from infected blankets, from wearing

other people's clothes, especially underwear or bathing trunks, and from intercourse. Both cause itching and scratching, particularly when warm at night. They are not dangerous and are very easy to treat with creams and lotions applied to the skin.

SYPHILIS

This is one of the oldest of the venereal diseases, formerly known as the pox. Before the discovery of penicillin, syphilis was a killer disease but fortunately now, so long as it is diagnosed, it is eminently curable and is in fact a very rare condition these days.

There are three stages to syphilis. The first to show is the development of a sore, called a chancre, which may occur anywhere on the genital organs from the tip of the penis to the inside of the vagina right up on the cervix. Chancres have been found on the nipples, the anus, and any part of the skin where there has been a cut or where the skin is very thin indeed. Chancres do disappear if they are left alone but they disappear far quicker if they are treated with penicillin by injection. Occasionally the sore appears for the first time on the lips, particularly if an infected partner has bitten his or her partner when he has the syphilis germ, called the spirochaete, in the mouth. There are millions of spirochaetes in the fluid on the sores. Seen under the microscrope, they are like very small, very fast-moving spiral rods.

The second stage of syphilis only comes if the chancre is not treated adequately. The spirochaetes spread from the first contact point, usually weeks after the intercourse that has caused the transmission of the disease, in fact anything from between two and eight months after. The patient may feel generally ill or run down, have a sore throat, be feverish, feel heavy, have a headache and come out in an unusual rash in any part of the body. Lymph nodes may also swell up at the tops of the thighs or in the armpits or the back of the neck. There may be some inflammation of the eyes.

The only safe way to diagnose for certain whether this state is due to syphilis is by a blood test, the TPHA (treponema pallida haemagglutination) test and the VDRL (the Venereal Disease Reference Laboratory) test.

It used to be quite common to see the third stage of syphilis, which affected the nervous system, or the heart, or the blood vessels from the heart; but nowadays this is very, very rare.

In a red light district, up to 1 percent of all the prostitutes are found to have positive syphilis tests. Some of them have inheritied the illness from their parents in which case they cannot transmit it further, as they do not have active germs in their body. Others may have acquired the illness by sexual contact even years previously, but if so the germs in their blood will always respond to treatment.

Syphilis can be transmitted from a mother to her unborn child and that is why, in almost all antenatal clinics in the UK, it is still routine to test for syphilis and to make sure that it cannot be handed on. If the blood test shows positive, treatment with penicillin is given for a few days and the baby is completely protected from the disease. Penicillin never harmed any unborn baby. If children *are* born with inherited syphilis, as they still are in some countries where penicillin is not easily available, they are often, if they survive at all, mentally backward, and there usually are other abnormalities; sometimes they are stillborn.

TRICHOMONAS

This condition, which occasionally gives rise to urethritis in men and women, also causes an inflammation in the vagina. It is common and is easily treated with Flagyl. The symptoms in women are a frothy, yellow, smelly discharge which dries yellow or green on underwear, accompanied by irritation, making the woman want to scratch. Diagnosis is easy for the doctor to make because of the vaginal discharge. It is, however, wrong for doctors just to diagnose and treat trichomonas without looking for other infections, because it is very common to have more than one STD at a time: for instance, gonorrhoea is found in about one in every four or five women who have had a trichomonas infection.

6
WHAT TO DO IF
YOU THINK YOU ARE PREGNANT OR
YOU THINK YOU HAVE AN STD

PREGNANCY

If you think you are pregnant and you want the baby, all you have to do in the first place to prepare yourself for the rest of the pregnancy and for the delivery is to go to your doctor, who will either undertake the antenatal care himself or refer you to a hospital. In any case he will almost certainly refer you to a hospital for the birth. Increasingly now, GPs are sharing antenatal care with hospitals, but there are still some hospital antenatal clinics that carry out all the care the mother-to-be needs.

If you do not want the baby, again go to your doctor, and, if he agrees, ask him to refer you to a hospital for a termination of pregnancy. If he does not agree, you can still have a termination by going to an advisory centre (see pages 95–101) or by arranging to see the Sister in the gynaecological clinic of your local district hospital. She may then tell you how you can be referred to the gynaecologist without going through your own doctor, though most hospitals do insist on a letter from the GP.

If you and your partner cannot make up your minds whether to keep the baby or not, for whatever reason, then you need counselling. The best people to help you make up your mind should be your own mother or close older relative, who will have to support you emotionally during the pregnancy and probably during the baby's childhood. It is not fair to take on this responsibility without letting them share it with you.

All the clinics that carry out terminations of pregnancy do have counsellors who can advise whether this is a good idea for you or not. There is seldom any great rush for the pregnancy to be terminated. Everyone can ask for a week to think it over and to discuss it with a trained counsellor or with some other expert. The addresses at the back of this book will give you access to the information you need. By and large, discussing the matter with your own friends is not as helpful as discussing it with professionals who have seen many, many cases before.

STD SYMPTOMS

The one symptom that is common to most sexually transmitted diseases is a discharge. In men the discharge comes from the tip of the penis down the urethra, and in women from the vagina and urethra.

The urethra, both in women and men, should not have discharges from it. So, if a man has a discharge he really has to start thinking whether he might have caught something, and he should seek medical advice. A discharge from the vagina is quite common, particularly in the middle of the monthly cycle. So a little clear discharge from the vagina is absolutely normal. If a woman has a discharge different from her normal losses, then she may very well want to seek medical advice. Discharges that smell or that stain underwear yellow or brown are quite reasonably worrying.

The first person to go to is your family doctor. Many young people, however, are worried that if their parents go to the same doctor, somehow or other they will get to hear of a son or daughter attending. Please try to go to your local doctor if there is any reason whatever to worry about the risk of having caught something.

If you cannot go to your GP the next best thing is to go to a clinic for genito-urinary medicine (GUM). All big hospitals in all towns have these clinics, and so does every one of the big district hospitals. Ask at the enquiry office for 'the clinic for genito-urinary medicine'. The clinic entrance is usually discreetly out of the way of the main entrances or corridors of the hospital.

Confidentiality in these clinics is enormously strict. Nobody can find out anything about any other patient by enquiry or by chance. Even I, as a doctor, wanted quite recently to let the staff of one GUM know that one of their patients had come to see me the day after she had been to the clinic, and that I had found something I thought had been missed which it was very important for the patient to have treated. The patient, who happened to be a prostitute, had a clinic telephone number which was totally confidential. I rang and asked to speak to one of the doctors but was told very pointedly that I could not do so, as they would not admit that the patient with me was a patient of theirs.

When I insisted that I really had some vital information that might save the patient's life, a second person came to the phone and told me rather rudely that confidentiality in their clinic was essential and that they could not divulge any information. I had not asked for anything to be divulged and I said I would be very upset indeed, and so would the patient who was sitting beside me, if I could not speak to a doctor. Eventually I was asked for my name and number and it was agreed that a doctor would phone me back. I am quite certain that both my name and number were checked to be sure that I was genuinely a doctor. Fifteen minutes later a doctor rang my surgery and was grateful that we were able to exchange information, as a result of which the patient was immediately admitted to hospital.

That is the degree of security that surrounds the running of a GUM clinic. Nothing is disclosed to anyone, not even a family doctor ringing on behalf of one of his patients, unless the clinic has checked on the person ringing, and is satisfied that any admission, or exchange of information, is absolutely essential as a life-saving measure for the patient. And they will still only do it with the patient's permission.

The tests that are carried out in the clinic consist of a general examination, an examination under a microscope of the discharges present, and blood tests. Sometimes the germs in the swabs have to be cultured in the laboratory, and this may take a day or two. Sometimes a few days are also required to find out what the blood tests show. Culturing the tests will show the doctors what antibiotics, if any, are needed to cure the condition. So it is worth waiting two days and going back to the clinic for the results, even if the discharge seems to have cleared itself. Something nasty may still be lurking and it may be possible to infect a new partner or re-infect one's old friend.

If you are asked to go back to the clinic for the results, please do go back. It is important.

Contact tracing

One of the reasons why diseases such as syphilis are being eliminated is because contacts of patients known to suffer from it are being traced efficiently and very tactfully.

It is much more important to trace somebody suffering from syphilis or AIDS than somebody who has a non-specific infection (NSU), when no definite germ has been isolated.

Untreated syphilis can be a killer disease, so it is important that if sufferers have the slightest idea from whom they may have caught it, they should ensure that the contact is also treated.

There are two overriding reasons for this. The first is to save the life of the person who has transmitted the disease. The second is to prevent further transmission to other people.

The patient being treated is given a contact card. The only information on this card is a code used in GUMs all over the country for a particular infection. For instance, A1 could be gonorrhoea (it is not) and so on. If a man has had intercourse with, say, three people, any one of whom might have given him his infection, he is given three cards to hand on to them. He should try to ensure that they go for a check-up. Of course, not everybody is aware of the identity of the person who has given them an infection, but that is quite rare.

If the contacts refuse to go for a check-up after being given a card – perhaps they cannot believe anything is wrong, or perhaps, selfishly, they could not care less, since they themselves do not notice they have anything wrong – further pressure may be brought to bear if the patient asks a nurse or social worker attached to the clinic, known as a contact tracer, to seek out the contact person.

7
CONCLUSIONS AND THE FUTURE

1987 brought about a unique happening: for the first time ever the Government spent tens of millions of pounds on advertisements and on putting leaflets concerning sexual practices into everybody's homes, and urging sensible precautions. The need for them to spend all this money and effort arose from the fear that an epidemic of AIDS would sweep through the country, as indeed it still may.

The freedom of the 1960s really did not bring much more happiness, although it certainly sexually liberated large numbers of young people – because of the pill, because in 1967 termination of pregnancy became widely available legally, and because a little later homosexual acts by consenting adults became legal. But in spite of the easy availability of safe and effective contraception, since the 1960s over 100,000 girls and older women each year have had a pregnancy terminated legally, and the numbers attending the genito-urinary medicine clinics has also steadily risen year by year. More than half the pregnancy terminations in the UK are still carried out in private charity clinics rather than on the National Health Service, which has not adequately fulfilled its role in this direction.

It is not possible to define promiscuity for either sex, since what is normal for one person may be too little, or may be excessive, for another. But it is possible to come to some conclusions about STDs, simply from medical evidence. And now we have entered a new era of the sexually transmitted disease. With AIDS, the whole community is threatened. So will all this publicity help to change people's habits?

Certainly it will in the 'straight' community. There is apparently already far less promiscuity and certainly far less unprotected vaginal intercourse with many partners than there used to be, even in the early 1980s. What will happen to the gay community?

Homosexual men have reacted in three ways to the warnings given about AIDS. Some have drastically cut down their number of partners and no longer frequent gay venues, picking up perhaps two or three partners in one evening, and certainly no longer have sex in any form unprotected by a condom. Some have continued exactly as before. And some have reacted in a perhaps surprising way: they have actually increased their numbers of partners with no apparent precautions. It seems likely that either some infected gays, for the time being at any rate, have the intention of taking as many people with them as they can, or that consciously or not there has been some yielding to a despairing instinct very closely akin to a suicidal act.

Will there be positive gains from a lessening in promiscuity? Certainly there will. Prostitution will not go away, of course, but there will be less rushing from partner to partner because of failure to obtain something exciting, satisfying and self-enhancing. People are genuinely frightened and probably slightly more careful about going into new relationships with full vaginal or anal intercourse even using a condom. So deeper and more rewarding relationships will grow when people look with more understanding for what they can give in terms of friendship. Friendship and emotional attachment can take a long time to develop, maybe a very long time. In the end, the physical side of a relationship is less important than the friendship. The sexual counter-revolution which is coming may bring more real happiness than the sexual revolution did.

But, above all, it is unthinkable that the medical profession and the pharmaceutical industry will fail to come up either with a vaccine against AIDS or even, in time, a cure for it.

As this is being written, a test for the AIDS virus is being perfected which will mean that doctors do not have to wait two or three months for an antibody to develop in the infected person's blood. So, earlier diagnosis means less risk of passing on the disease. Doubtless, too, the AIDS research will produce treatments to benefit sufferers from other chronic diseases, so medicine as a whole will have advanced more quickly.

APPENDICES

PREGNANCY ADVISORY BUREAUX

Telephone	Address
021 643 0644	**Birmingham Pregnancy Consultation Service** 14–16 Temple Street Birmingham B2 5BG
0253 23009	**Blackpool Pregnancy Testing and Counselling Centre** Stanley Buildings 3 Caunce Street Blackpool
0256 53129	**British Pregnancy Advisory Service** Basingstoke Branch Church Grange Health Centre Bramleys Drive Basingstoke RG21 1QN
021 643 1461	**British Pregnancy Advisory Service** Birmingham Branch Guildhall Buildings Navigation Street Birmingham B2 4BT
0202 28762	**British Pregnancy Advisory Service** Bournemouth (Dean Park) Branch 23 Ophir Road Bournemouth
0202 228762	**British Pregnancy Advisory Service** Bournemouth (Pelhams) Branch Pelhams Clinic Millhams Road Bournemouth

0273 509726   **British Pregnancy Advisory Service**
Brighton Branch
Wistons Site
Chatsworth Road
Brighton
Sussex BN1 5PA

0244 27113   **British Pregnancy Advisory Service**
Chester Branch
98A Foregate Street
Chester CH1 1HB

0482 23777   **British Pregnancy Advisory Service**
Coventry Branch
Coundon Health Clinic
Barker Butts Land
Coventry

0302 4893   **British Pregnancy Advisory Service**
Doncaster Branch
The Bungalow
1A Avenue Road
Doncaster
South Yorkshire

0482 223944   **British Pregnancy Advisory Service**
Hull Branch
32 Beverley Road
Hull HU3 1YF

0203 597344   **British Pregnancy Advisory Service**
Leamington Spa Branch
Holly Walk
Leamington Spa
Warwickshire

0532 443861   **British Pregnancy Advisory Service**
Leeds Branch
8 The Headrow
Leeds
Yorkshire

051 227 3721   **British Pregnancy Advisory Service**
Liverpool Branch
20–22 Rodney Street
Liverpool L1 2TQ

01 222 0985   **British Pregnancy Advisory Service**
London Branch
7 Belgrave Road
London SW1

0582 26287   **British Pregnancy Advisory Service**
Luton Branch
3A Upper George Street
Luton LU1 2QY

061 236 7777   **British Pregnancy Advisory Service**
Manchester Branch
Suite F, Ground Floor
Fourways House
57 Hilton Street
Manchester M1 2EJ

0234 46574   **British Pregnancy Advisory Service**
Milton Keynes Branch
First Floor
Eaglestones Health Centre
Standing Way
Milton Keynes MK6 5AZ

0742 738326   **British Pregnancy Advisory Service**
Sheffield Branch
160 Charles Street
Sheffield S1 2NE

0793 30366   **British Pregnancy Advisory Service**
Swindon Branch
Priory Road Health Clinic
Priory Road
Swindon SN3 2EZ

0602 621450   **East Midland Pregnancy Advisory Service**
The Grange
1 Private Road
Sherwood
Nottingham

01 434 4235/
01 487 3991   **The Gerrard Street Clinic**
36 Gerrard Street
London W1V 7LP

01 207 4792   **London Youth Advisory Centre**
26 Prince of Wales Road
London NW5

01 452 7646   **Marie Stopes North London PAB**
65 Shoot-up Hill
London NW2

061 450 4191/
3336   **Marie Stopes Manchester**
1 Police Street
Manchester M2 7LQ

0532 440685   **Marie Stopes Centre**
10 Queens Square
Leeds 2

01 580 4847/
8/9   **Metropolitan Pregnancy Control Centre**
77 Tottenham Court Road
London W1

0253 29096   **Pregnancy Advisory Service Blackpool**
93A Bingdon Street
Blackpool FY1 1PP

01 637 8962   **Pregnancy Advisory Service London**
11/13 Charlotte Street
London W1

051 236 8668   **Pregnancy Advisory Service
Liverpool**
Fourth Floor
Hepworth Chambers
Church Street
Liverpool L1 3BG

**061 228 1887/
8**   **Pregnancy Advisory Service
Manchester**
5th Floor
Newton Buildings
Newton Street
Manchester M1 2EJ

0782 632784   **Pregnancy Advisory Service
Newcastle-upon-Lyme**
1A George Street
Newcastle-upon-Lyme
Staffordshire

01 891 3173   **Pregnancy Advisory Service
Twickenham**
Rosslyn
17 Rosslyn Road
East Twickenham
Middlesex TW1 2AR

01 437 7125   **Pregnancy and Gynaecological
Advisory Service**
26 Fouberts Place
London W1N 1HG

01 580 9001   **Preterm**
40 Mortimer Street
London W1N 7RB

0742 730990   **Sheffield Pregnancy and Counselling
Service**
276 Glossop Road
Sheffield S10 5HL

0482 23777   **Sister Rose Pregnancy Advisory Centre (Hull)**
139 Beverley Road
Hull

0532 456914   **Sister Rose Pregnancy Advisory Centre (Leeds)**
4 Albion Street
Leeds 1

0902 21131   **Sister Rose Pregnancy Advisory Centre (Wolverhampton)**
Second Floor
19–21 Queen Street
Wolverhampton

061 834 0440   **Sister Rose Pregnancy Advisory Centre (Manchester)**
Fifth Floor
2 St John Street
Manchester 3

01 388 0622   **The Well Woman Centre**
Marie Stopes House
108 Whitefield Street
London W1

01 388 4843   **The Well Woman Centre**
114 Whitefield Street
London W1

0742 662341   **Young Peoples Consultation Centre Ltd**
408 Ecclesall Road
Sheffield S11 8PJ

SCOTLAND

The registration of these Bureaux is a matter for the Secretary of State for Scotland.

Glasgow

041 204 1832 — **British Pregnancy Advisory Service**
245 North Street (2nd Floor)
Charing Cross
Glasgow G3 7DL

041 221 9042 — **Sister Rose Pregnancy Advisory Centre**
Fourth Floor
42 St Enoch Square
Glasgow G1

WALES

The registration of this Bureaux is a matter for the Secretary of State for Wales.

Cardiff

0222 372389 — **British Pregnancy Advisory Service**
4 High Street Arcade Chambers
Cardiff

FAMILY PLANNING ASSOCIATION CLINICS

(courtesy of The FPA, 27 Mortimer Street, London W1 7RS)

Telephone	Clinic address	NHS or Private
0256 26980	**Basingstoke FPA Clinic** 8 Fairfields Road Basingstoke, Hampshire *Birth control, all methods, psychosexual and menopausal advice, well-woman, pregnancy testing, youth advisory service free*	Private
0234 62436	**Bedford FPA Clinic** 38b St Peters Street, Bedford *Psycho-sexual advice*	Private
021 454 0236	**Birmingham FPA Clinic** 7 York Road, Birmingham *Menopause*	Private
0202 38741	**Cardiff FPA Clinic** Ante-Natal Clinic Suite University Hospital of Wales Heath Park, Cardiff	Private
0228 36451	**Carlisle FPA Clinic** Central Clinic 50 Victoria Place, Carlisle	Private

| 0203 543514 | **Coventry FPA Clinic** Stoke Aldermoor Aldermoor Lane, Coventry CU3 1BN | **Private** |

| 0632 783811 | **Gateshead FPA Clinic** Queen Elizabeth's Hospital Out-patients Dept Gateshead, Tyne & Wear | **Private (NHS for selected patients)** |

| 0494 26666 | **High Wycombe FPA Clinic** 6 Harlow Road High Wycombe *Birth control, menopause advice, youth advisory service, well-woman, pregnancy testing* | **Private** |

| 0624 833464 | **Isle of Man (Castletown) FPA Clinic** Janets Corner, Castletown *Birth control* | **Private (free for certain patients)** |

| 0624 23526 | **Isle of Man (Douglas)** Noble's Isle of Man Hospital Westmoreland Road, Douglas *Birth control, all methods* | **Private (free for certain patients)** |

| — | **Isle of Man (Douglas) FPA Clinic** The School Clinic Murrays Road Douglas *Birth control* | **Private (free for certain patients)** |

| 0624 813952 | **Isle of Man (Ramsey)** Ramsey Cottage Hospital Ramsey *Birth control* | **Private (free for certain patients)** |

| 0563 25288 | **Kilmarnock FPA Clinic** | Private |

| 0482 29360 | **Kingston upon Hull FPA Clinic** *Birth control, all methods, well-woman, menopausal advice* | Private |

| 0234 62436 | **Luton FPA Clinic** Liverpool Road Health Centre Luton, Bedfordshire | Private |

| 0603 52244 Ext 149 | **Newport FPA Clinic** | Private (NHS Gwent patients only) |

| 0602 47043 | **Nottingham FPA Clinic** *Birth control, all methods, well-woman, pregnancy testing* | Private |

| 0742 21191 | **Sheffield FPA Clinic** 17 North Church Street Sheffield *Menopausal advice, sub-fertility, research in dysmenorrhoea, premenstral tension syndrome, birth control, menopausal treatment* | Private |

| 01 602 2723 | **Shepherds Bush FPA Clinic** *Birth control, all methods, pregnancy testing, counselling* *Menopausal advice, psycho-sexual counselling* | NHS

Private |

| — | **Southend FPA Clinic** Kent Elms Clinic Rayleigh Road Eastwood, Essex | Private |

0234 **62436**	**St Albans FPA Clinic** Out-patients Dept, Mid Herts Wing City Hospital, Church Crescent St Albans, Hertfordshire	**Private**
—	**Sunderland FPA Clinic** The General Hospital Out-patients Dept Chester Road, Sunderland	**Private** **(NHS for** **selected** **patients,** **Durham** **only)**
0892 **30002**	**Tunbridge Wells FPA Clinic** 21 Dudley Road Tunbridge Wells, Kent *Birth control, all methods, psycho-* *sexual and menopausal advice*	**Private**

While many of the Family Planning Association clinics whose addresses are given on the previous pages will look after young people, the Brook Advisory Centres specialize in offering free birth control advice and supplies to young people. They were started in 1964 by Helen Brook. They are for boys as much as girls, and young couples who can either come together or alone, or come with a friend for company.

They are absolutely free. All the conversations are absolutely private and there is complete confidentiality. Most are open full time, evenings and Saturday mornings. It is advisable, but not absolutely essential, to telephone or write to the nearest centre to find out exactly when they are open and when they are closed.

Birmingham
021 455 0491   **Brook Advisory Centre**
9 York Road
Birmingham B16 9HX

021 643 5341   **City Centre Brook**
Top Floor, 8–10 Albert Street
Birmingham B4 7UD

021 554 7553   **Handsworth Brook Centre**
102 Hamstead Road, Handsworth
Birmingham B19 1DG

021 328 4544   **Saltley Brook Centre**
3 Washwood Heath Road
Saltley, Birmingham B8 1SH

Bristol
0272 736657   **Brook Advisory Centre (Avon)**
21 Richmond Hill, Clifton
Bristol BS8 1BA

Coventry
0203 412627 for   **Gynaecological Out-patients**
appointments   Coventry and Warwickshire Hospital
Stoney Stanton Road, Coventry

Edinburgh
031 229 3596   **Brook Advisory Centre**
2 Lower Gilmore Place (Office)
50 Gilmore Place (Centre)
Edinburgh EH3 9NY

Merseyside
051 709 4558   **Brook Look-In**
9 Gambier Terrace
Liverpool L17BG

London
—   **Barnsbury Centre**
Barnsbury Clinic
Carnegie Street
London N1 9QW

01 274 4995	**Brixton Brook Centre** 53 Acre Lane London SW2 5TN
01 323 1522 for enquiries 01 580 2991 for appoint- ments	**Brook Advisory Centre** 233 Tottenham Court Road London W1P 9AE
01 272 5599	**Islington Brook Centre** 6–9 Manor Gardens off Holloway Road London N7 6LA
01 703 9660/ 7880	**Kennington Brook Centre** Moffat Health Centre, 65 Sancroft Street, off Kennington Road, London SE11 5NG
01 703 9660/ 7880	**Lewisham Brook Centre** Lewisham Hospital, Ante-Natal Dept. Lewisham High Street London SE13 6LH
—	**Newham Centre** West Ham Lane Clinic 84 West Ham Lane, Stratford London E15 4PT
01 580 2991	**Shoreditch Brook Centre** 210 Kingsland Road London E2 8EB
01 703 9660/ 7880	**Stockwell Brook Centre** Rose McAndrew Community Health Service Clinic Beale House, Lingham Street London SW9

01 703 9660/ 7880	**Walworth Brook Centre** 153a East Street, Walworth London SE17 2SD
01 703 9660/ 7880	**Wandsworth Centre** St Christopher's Health Centre Wheeler Court, Plough Road London SW11 2AY

Where to go if you have any problems about your ability to perform sexually.

The Association of Sexual and Marital Therapists
P.O. Box 62
Sheffield S10 3TS

who have a list of sex therapists who work along Masters and Johnson's methods.

The Institute of Psychosexual Medicine
11 Chandos Street
Cavendish Square
London W1M 9DE

who have a list of counsellors on psychosexual matters all over the UK.

National Marriage Guidance Council
Little Church Street
Rugby CV21 3AP

for a list of clinics which specialize in counselling for marital sexual therapy.

Since about 10 percent to 15 percent of all people have some kind of homosexual tendency, whether male or female, and may have worries about it, here are some useful addresses and telephone numbers in London to which people may turn for very friendly advice and information on centres more local to their area.

01 981 2717 01 980 7222 0345 581151	**Healthline Telephone Service** *For 24-hour service recorded information on AIDS. For calls from outside London, the 0345 number will be charged at local rates.*
01 407 1010	**The Haemophiliac Society** PO Box 9 16 Trinity Street, London SE1 1DE *(Advice for haemophiliacs and their partners.)*
Helpline 01 833 2971	**Terrence Higgins Trust** BM/AIDS London WC1N 3XX Mon–Fri 7pm–10pm Sat–Sun 3pm–10pm *(This is particularly helpful for gays and lesbians who are frightened they may have caught a sexually transmitted disease, in particular AIDS.)*
01 359 7371	**London Friend** 274 Upper Street, London N1
01 837 7324	**London Lesbian and Gay Switchboard**
01 227 4413	**Portobello Project** 49 Porchester Road, London W2 *(This project particularly helps gay men aged 14–21.)*
01 430 2341	**SCODA (Standing Conference on Drug Abuse)** 1–4 Hatton Place, London EC1N 8MD

FURTHER READING

The Joy of Sex by Alex Comfort (Quartet Books, 1974)
The Technique of Sex by Anthony Havil (Thorsons Publishers Ltd, 6th edition 1983)